NOT A TOTAL WASTE

By

B.M. LLOYD

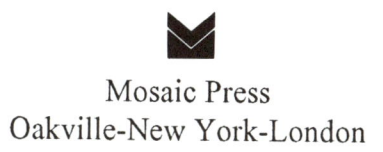

Mosaic Press
Oakville-New York-London

Canadian Cataloguing in Publication Data

Lloyd, B.M., 1936-
Not a total waste

ISBN 0-88962-540-9

1. AIDS (Disease) - Patients - Biography.
I. Title

RC607.A26L57 1993   362.1'969792'0092   C93-093482-2

No part of this book may be reproduced or transmitted in any form, by any means, electronic or mechanical, including photocopying and recording information storage and retrieval systems, without permission in writing from the publisher, except by a reviewer who may quote brief passages in a review.

Published by MOSAIC PRESS, P.O. Box 1032, Oakville, Ontario, L6J 5E9, Canada. Offices and warehouse at 1252 Speers Road, Units 1&2, Oakville, Ontario, L6L 5N9, Canada.

Mosaic Press acknowledges the assistance of the Canada Council and the Ontario Arts Council in support of its publishing programme.

Copyright © B.M. Lloyd, 1993
Design by Patty Gallinger
Typeset by Jackie Ernst

Printed and bound in Canada.

ISBN 0-88962-540-9 PB

MOSAIC PRESS:
In Canada:
    MOSAIC PRESS, 1252 Speers Road, Units 1&2, Oakville, Ontario L6L 5N9, Canada. P.O. Box 1032, Oakville, Ontario L6J 5E9
In the U.K.:
    John Calder (Publishers) Ltd., 9-15 Neal Street, London, WCZH 9TU, England.

DEDICATION

People with AIDS-related illnesses must contend with a lethal disease, in addition to legal and social oppression.

Their medical and personal caregivers experience disorders of burnout. Institutional churches do not always effectively stress the unprejudiced, spiritual comfort aspects of religion for the Gay and Lesbian Community. Scientists are still engaged in a determined fight against this destructive disease.

I dedicate this book in the memory of our only son, to all individuals with HIV/AIDS, and to those who battle on behalf of patients suffering from ANY death-threatening illness. May we continue to provide them with our nonjudgmental respect, our compassion and our support.

In order to provide assistance for people with AIDS and AIDS research, part of the money obtained from the sale of this book will be pledged to the Canadian Foundation for AIDS Research and the Fife House Foundation, which provides housing for AIDS patients.

To you, Michael, because you taught us how to live and to recognize the permanence of death. Your loved ones carry you in our hearts and minds, constantly.

WITH THANKS

This is a TRUE STORY, with names and places changed to provide privacy for those persons involved. I'm grateful to my husband, my daughter and her family for their patience throughout this therapeutic description of an AIDS-related illness and death. The support and confidence placed in me by Michael's friends was a powerful impetus behind my writing. This is their story, too. The love of my family and friends assisted me in my search for understanding of the loss of an only son, only brother and dear friend.

The potential value of this book as a reference source for others experiencing grief and facing a death-threatening illness, provided an essential driving force. If this book can prevent one person from risking their life with unsafe sex, or help one person to carry on after the death of a beloved, then it will have some merit.

Trusted friends assisted by proofreading many manuscript drafts. The Preface and Afterthoughts, provided with compassion and love, gave me needed initiative towards completion. This book would never have been written without the encouragement of loved ones, the confidence of authors, editors and publisher or the assurance of caring community activists.

Over seven hundred years ago, this beautiful prayer was written by Saint Francis of Assisi. It must have nourished others at that time, in the same manner as it has helped Michael's loved ones to cope with his loss.

"Lord, make me an instrument of Thy Peace.
Where there is hatred, let me sow love.
Where there is injury, pardon.
Where there is doubt, faith.
Where there is despair, hope.
Where there is darkness, light.
Where there is sadness, joy.
O Divine Master, grant that I may not so much seek to be consoled, as to console; to be understood, as to understand; to be loved, as to love; for it is in giving that we receive, it is in pardoning that we are pardoned, and it is in dying that we are born to Eternal Life".

TABLE OF CONTENTS

Preface/June Callwood	ix
Section One	1
Section Two	66
Section Three	169
Aftermath	213
Afterthoughts	281
Tables	283
Rubbers and Romance	285
Tasks to be Completed After the Death	287
Music Sources	289
Organizations and Support Groups	291
Glossary	299
Bibliography	304
AIDS Charts	320

PREFACE

As anyone who has been through it knows, there is no pain on earth to compare with the death of one's child. A woman whose daughter was killed in a car accident ten years ago recently learned that she has cancer. She was heard to murmur, "Terminal cancer is not the worst thing that can happen in a lifetime." When bereaved parents meet and accidentally discover the terrible loss they have in common, they are stricken into silence. One makes a helpless gesture, the other shrugs in sorrowful acknowledgement, and they change the subject. There are no words for a grief so deep and lasting.
    The woman who wrote this book about the death of her son from AIDS is not using her real name--or his--but her agony is genuine. As her son's illness approached its final ravaging stage, his body beginning to shred, it became clear that he didn't want to be moved from the apartment he loved. He wished instead to stay among possessions he had acquired over the years, in his own bed, rather than be transported to the vagaries of an impersonal hospital room. Such a plan would have been unthinkable only a few years ago, but not any more. The Annals of General Internal Medicine in 1992 confirmed that 73 percent of people, given the choice, would prefer to die at home. Institutions increasingly are seen as inappropriate places for most deaths, and even for most births. Consequently the delivery of health services is undergoing a massive shift from hospitals to the community; home care almost everywhere in Canada is increasingly expert and available.

The young man in this story was not so fortunate as to have all the professional support he needed, but he had his mother. She nursed him tenderly and faithfully, and they shared the sanity of laughter. She was beside him, holding him, when he stopped breathing.

The story is the triumph of two brave people. They could not defeat death but they gave it a great fight. Mother and son reached inside themselves and found strengths they didn't know they possessed; when their courage faltered, they comforted one another. NOT A TOTAL WASTE is about what Philippe Aries calls "a tame death"--a death cushioned against horror by love. It is about deathless bonds between parent and child, the gallant spirit of a dying youth, and the grit of an indomitable mother.

--June Callwood

SECTION ONE

CHAPTER ONE

The grandchildren, Sean and Jenni, usually share the summer with us in Northwestern Ontario. It removes them from the heat of the city, and allows them to participate in local swimming and sailing lessons. More importantly, it gives us an opportunity to spoil them rotten and then send them back to their loving parents. They had arrived on the last Friday in JUNE, 1990. It was time for them to depart for their first swimming lesson early Monday morning, when the phone rang. I stumbled over the strewn Sunday newspapers to grab it first.

"Hello".

"Maria, it's Penny. Michael's very sick. There's a bad smell coming from his room. He kept the TV set on all night, and he's not answering when I knock on his bedroom door. I think that you'd better come down."

"I guess that I knew he would get worse, Penny, but I thought we had more time. How long has this been going on? When I visited with him two weeks ago, he seemed in pretty good shape."

"I've been away all week-end. He drove to Montreal with Lucy and Therese to visit at her family's cottage. When I saw him last Thursday, he didn't seem quite right. Michael was sort of distant, and didn't respond when I spoke to him. He merely sat in front of his stereo listening to music and stared at me. I assumed that he was just tired."

"What is the bad smell? Vomit? Excretion?"

NOT A TOTAL WASTE

"I don't know. I was running late this morning and when he didn't answer, I didn't open his door."
"Oh God, Penny. Is he alive?"
"That's why I called. He won't answer the phone. I'm calling from work. You'd better come down."
"Okay. I'll get out on the next plane. I appreciate you letting me know. I'll see you to-night."

When I hung up, I realized that the grandchildren and Bruce, my husband, were standing at the top of the stairs, quietly listening. They were watching my face intently.

"What's the matter with Uncle Mike, Nana?" Sean asked.
"Why do you have to fly down, Nana?" querried Jenni.
"It's bad, is it?" from my husband, Bruce.
"It sounds like it. I'll have to leave right away. Penny says that his room smells, and that he won't answer when she knocks on the door, or phones. Michael could be already dead."
"See if you can get out this morning. I'll take the kids down to the pool and get right back. Get packed--I'll drive you to the airport."

The plane left our small city shortly after ten that morning, and I arrived at Michael's apartment in Toronto's Cabbagetown just after twelve. Usually, when I put my key in the lock, there was a feeling of exhilaration and expectation. Our joy at seeing one another and the unique rapport we shared made every visit special. Ever since Michael had been a little boy, we would both get caught up in an idea, and pass thoughts back and forth at lightening speed-- rarely, if ever, completing a sentence, and yet grasping concepts effectively. Spontaneous, rapid-fire chatter seemed to be the rule. Sharing the love of art, music, theatre and good food made each visit an adventure. Michael had lived and studied in many parts of the world, and this was mirrored in his selection of various restaurants in Toronto. He'd ask which country we'd like to eat in that night-- determine an ethnic selection, and we'd jump in a cab. More recently, he'd felt too nauseated to eat much, but we'd still give it a try. Italian pasta and fish seemed to be his favourite things lately, and the waiter at his favourite bistro took delight in seeing him.

This morning I entered the apartment and was met by an empty silence, enforced with the sickening-sweet stench of diarrhea. I shut the door softly and leaned against it, my head reeling. I wanted to hear him sing out, "Hi Mom, I'm here. How was the trip?" I put down my flight bag and walked quietly down the hall towards his room. After gently tapping on his door, I opened it. Michael was sitting on the edge of his bed, holding onto the closest edge of his dresser. The stench hit me hard with the opening of the door, but the shock of seeing him so ill made my knees feel wobbly. I did my best to put on a grin, and said,

"Hi Mike. Penny phoned to say that she was concerned, so I came down. I thought that I'd surprise you. How do you like my new dress?"

I had bought a turquoise and white print two-piece outfit. I knew he would appreciate it. The mention of the dress had served as a ruse to divert attention away from Michael's state. I needed a few minutes to compose myself, and expected that Michael did, too. He always took a genuine interest in my apparel, and liked to see me make an effort in taking care of myself. My weight often fluctuated too much, and he cautioned me on my health. If I let my hair style go, he'd make appointments for me with his friend Bob, who had been the Artistic Director at a top Toronto salon before he opened his own shop. "Take care of yourself, Mom. Remember that there are no guarantees. Life's a complicated game. It's just one great crapshoot, Ma," had been one of Michael's speculations. Patiently, I confirmed my determination to remain vital by my use of seat belts, absention from smoking, continued regimen of exercises and sincere efforts to stabilize my weight. Now there he sat, weakened and dehydrated from a secondary infection that caused fever, forceful vomiting and violent diarrhea.

I looked closely and noticed that his feet and legs had turned a bluish colour, up past his knees. His face was damp and fever-flushed. Michael's eyes were having trouble focusing on mine. The panic I felt made it difficult to regulate my breathing. With an effort, I spoke calmly. I said,

"What can I get for you, son? Do you need help to get to the toilet?"
He muttered, "No, Ma. I just need to have something to drink".
"Okay, how about some juice? I'll get it for you, and then I'll get changed and tackle the rest".

"No, Ma, just some Coke. There's some in the fridge. Everything else makes me barf."

He sipped the cold fluid and then lay back down against the pillows. A little smile touched his thin face, and he closed his eyes. No wonder Penny had sounded more irritated than concerned, when she had called. She was probably very frightened. She and Michael had known each other since high school, and had been room-mates in Ottawa where they both studied. After Penny completed Teacher's College and gained employment in Toronto, they had shared this apartment. It was to have been a temporary measure until she had relocated herself, but she had remained there for two years. They understood one another well, enjoyed each other's companionship and some mutual friendships. They had weathered the emotional ups and downs of study and work related stress better than most people. Theirs was a supportive alliance, devoid of any sexual relationship. Penny had her personal goals, and accepted Michael's homosexual life-style.

I changed into jeans and a shirt, and stood at Michael's bedroom door. Even though the early July morning was already oppressively hot and humid, he lay with his favourite jade-green duvet over his still form. His bedroom window was opened approximately a hand-span in height, but his white drapes were tightly drawn. Neither light nor street sounds seemed to penetrate the room. The hall light illuminated his pale face and flushed cheeks. His eyes were shut, and he rested against three pillows tucked behind his back.

"Michael, are you awake? Do you want me to get you something else to drink?" No response. God, please let him live. Please. Answer me, Michael. Please. I moved slowly towards his bed and sat down. The strength that had driven me to this place now seemed to have gone. I could feel a sort of trembling take over my legs and hands. "Mike, honey, please wake up. Do you want me to call your doctor?" It was all that I could trust myself to say.

He stirred just slightly. "Mom, I'm just tired. I'll be fine. I can't drink anything else right now. It makes me puke. Sorry."

"I could make you clear tea, dear. But that can wait. Will you let me take your temperature right now? Then I'll call your doctor, just to inform him about your illness."

He squiggled down into the bed a bit, turned his face towards his bedside clock, and then slowly faced me.

"What day is this, Mom? When did you come?"

I told him that it was Monday, and inserted the thermometer into his mouth. When it beeped, it read 104.7 degrees Fahrenheit.

I left the room silently and called his doctor from the other telephone in the dining room. It was hard to control my emotions. I explained to the receptionist that it was essential that Michael's doctor call me as soon as he was free. She explained that he was out of town at a conference, but that he would call the next morning about eight o'clock. She suggested that I take Michael to the hospital immediately, but I demurred. I couldn't arrange that unless Michael agreed.

His frail appearance and lassitude was a heart breaking contrast to his alert and mischievous manner on my previous visit two weeks ago. Michael's deterioration had been rapid. The shock hit me hard. It seemed sensible to keep myself busy while he slept. I scoured the bathroom, washed the dishes, and sponge-mopped the floors in the rest of the apartment. After hastily unpacking the few clothes that I had brought, I tip-toed back to his room and peered at him.

"Mike, have you had any medication today?"
"I can't remember, Mom."
"How 'bout I get you some apple juice to take with your pills, and then I'll make tea for us. You need fluids to prevent dehydration, dear. Can you try?"
"Okay, Ma. But first, can you help me to get a shower?"
"Sure. We'll do that now."

I had not seen Michael naked since he was a tiny boy. His emaciated, gaunt appearance caused me to take a deep breath so that I would not cry out. He leaned on me only slightly, as he doggedly pushed one foot ahead of the other, lurching towards the bathroom. Once there, he insisted on taking care of himself, so I washed the glasses in the kitchen. Afterwards I darted into his room, to change his bedding. I turned on the fan and opened the window wide to alleviate the diarrhea stench, and rapidly sponged his floor. After

NOT A TOTAL WASTE

I had tidied up his dresser top, I lay out a large T-shirt to help absorb the perspiration caused by the fever.

Michael showered and crawled back into his bed. He was incontinent, no longer able to control his bowel or bladder, but I did not properly respond to these changes immediately. I had remembered to put plastic sheeting under his linens to protect the mattress from further accidents, but it was obvious that the mattress would need replacing. He sipped some apple juice with the many pills that he had pointed out to me from his dresser. It looked like a pharmacy, with at least twelve different bottles lined up in a row. I wanted to sweep them onto the floor with one movement. It made me angry that none of these had been sufficient to prevent this infection from attacking him.

Later that afternoon Michael woke up and asked for tea. When it was prepared, he put on his dressing gown and managed to come into the dining room and sit in his favourite chair. I had bought him an Obus form and chair pad to provide back support, and some cushioning for his tailbone. There was so very little flesh left on his bones, that it hurt him to sit for any length of time. When I teased him that this was his "handsome prince throne", he would give me that Michael look--a long, serious stare with his brows knotted together. After the tea, I leaned over and took his two thin hands in mine. He looked directly into my eyes, and I saw his pain. Neither of us could stop tears from spilling over and running down our cheeks.

"Michael, I love you so much. You know that. I'll do whatever you tell me. I just don't know what to do. Tell me what you want, dear. I will help you fight this thing, or I'll take you to Amsterdam where Euthanasia is legal. Just tell me what you want me to do."

He stared, with his eyes suddenly round. He gasped in shock, and more quickly than I thought feasible, got to his room. He did not shut the door, but lay across his bed. I buried my head in my hands and tried to pull myself together. I whimpered in pain. Oh, God forgive me. I did not mean to hurt him. I want him to live, if that's what he wants. He seems to have given up, and lost his will to survive. I want him to choose the quality of his life. I want to jolt him into confronting this illness, and force him to fight back. But why must he suffer like this? Why? Help me, God, to help him. Please.

I walked in, pulled the drapes together, and shut off the noisy fan. I eased him out of his housecoat and pulled the sheet over him. He sighed and stretched.

"Mom, my answer is that I want to live. Please Mom, help me."

"Okay, dear. We'll fight like hell. We'll wait for the doctor to get back to us in the morning, and then take it from there. Now just rest, Michael. If you need me, call me."

I huddled on the dining room futon, and wondered why I had pushed Michael for a life or death decision. My ignorance regarding Holland's policy, which prevents tourists from obtaining medical death-assistance, was apparent. It made sense that the patient must be known to the doctor for a long period of time, should he require assistance in ending his life. Naturally, no country wishes to become the world's suicide Mecca. Michael had stated his desire to live, and I was determined to help. Nevertheless, it hurt me to watch his painful suffering from this incurable disease. Ending a terminally-ill patient's suffering did not seem the same thing as "aiding and abetting the suicide" of an emotionally disturbed individual. As Michael's mother, my heart bled to see his heroics, despite such a demeaning lack of personal dignity. It was also logical that the laws remain sufficiently stringent to protect against the abuse of euthanasia. The anguish remained. I had no answers.

When Penny came home from work about two hours later, Michael was still asleep. She asked me if the doctor had been called. I explained that he was unavailable until the following morning, but we'd cope until then. She willingly shopped for more fruit juices and some adult-sized diapers. Later I overheard her on the phone, talking to Lucy and Therese.

When she hung up, she walked into Michael's room and said, "Hey lazy-bones, get up. We're going to Lucy's for chicken dinner, remember?" I froze in shock. How could she possibly imagine that he could get out of the bed? His fever was down to 101 degrees now, but in his weakened condition he should just rest and take fluids. His response was feeble, but clear.

NOT A TOTAL WASTE

"Oh, I guess that I forgot. Pass me my jeans and shirt from behind the door. Ask Mom to get ready, too."

I had been reading the Globe and Mail, and wondered if I could get up from the table. Penny stood watching me. I asked, "Do you really think that this is a good idea?" She frowned, and walked back to her front room.

Somehow Michael dressed himself, the cab arrived, and we got to Lucy's apartment. The meal was beautifully prepared, and the bubbly chatter and laughter around the table was a delight. Michael spoke little, ate a small amount, and then stumbled to the bathroom with a violent attack of diarrhea. He was in the washroom about fifteen minutes, but it seemed like hours. Lucy left the table to check on him, and provided him with a clean pair of track pants and socks. He insisted that he was fine, and tried to rinse out his clothing in the sink. Therese and Penny were visibly upset when Lucy returned. Finishing supper was out of the question. We sat sipping on coffee, quietly lost in our own thoughts.

"I can't bear to see Michael diminished to this. The deterioration is extensive. Even his ability to reason seems impaired. This is one hell of a way for him to live," I said.

"Maria, don't even think that way. He has to keep trying. He can't give up," replied Lucy.

"I know what you mean about the quality of his life,
Maria. But don't hint at ending it. It's illegal, and could be misunderstood. It's got to be an infection that we can fight."

"God, I hope so. It tears me apart, seeing him lose control like this. He's so proud and dignified. Michael hates to be dependent upon anyone. I feel so helpless... and so angry at what is happening to him."

"Shush, he'll hear you. Call a cab and get him back home," stated Therese.

Penny spoke through the bathroom door to notify Michael that the cab had been ordered, and we were prepared to leave. He answered that he'd be right out. Once we had him home, he put on the diapers, drank a full glass of orange juice and fell into a deep sleep. I dozed intermittently, constantly checking on his breathing and fever. His temperature was still close to normal.

In the morning, Michael's friend David called around eight o'clock. I explained why I was back in Toronto, so soon after my previous visit. He said that he'd call later on to see if Michael was admitted to the hospital, and that he'd notify Corey and Ted. They were two more of Mike's closest friends. I appreciated David looking after those details, since I had no idea how to contact them.

Dr. Drake called promptly at eight thirty. When I explained the situation, he urged me to get Michael to the hospital as soon as possible. He would contact the medical team there, and would keep in touch through them. He asked me to call him immediately if I had any other concerns. His sincerity and support were so apparent that I discerned why Michael felt safe with him. He had been Michael's doctor since he had first been tested positively for the HIV virus in 1987.

After letting Michael know that we'd be leaving for the hospital, I helped him to take his medication, and stowed his vials of medication within my purse. At the last minute, he decided to have a shower, so I waited at the dining room table. In this way, I could be close enough for him to call me, if he required some assistance.

CHAPTER TWO

As I waited, I admired the beauty of the room. Bookcases lined two walls, overflowing with novels in several languages, art, architectural texts, research books, linguistic dictionaries, and teaching methodology books. Next to the large window, black shelving held all of his stereo equipment, records, CD's and tapes. The large black futon, on which I had slept, was underneath the window. On the opposite side stood an unpainted desk with his computer, printer and supplies.

As I sat there in the dining room, I sipped tea and reminisced about Michael's lifetime. Memories flickered like a documentary film, clearly and promptly through my mind. The colourful prints on the walls were from many parts of the world in which Michael had studied, lived and travelled. He had sanded down the old oaken floors and varnished them to a high gloss, and had reclaimed the oak trim around the doors. The walls were painted a deep marine blue, and the window blind was sparkling white. It was a beautiful, friendly room that hugged you when you entered. The entire apartment was efficiently organized and attractive.

From my vantage point, I could look directly into the kitchen. Glossy-white cupboards built by Michael were completed with black Italian tile counters. The six-foot high window looked onto the fresh green grass of the back yard. African violets and begonias bloomed upon the window sill over the stainless steel sink. The pine knife-holder, dustbuster, potholders and dish towels hung unobstrusively next to the grumbling old fridge. The blender, teapot and cannister set were all that remained on the glossy counters. The silver kettle, with the noisiest train whistle that I could locate, waited on the gas stove. It had been a surprise gift for him on my last trip, since he had worried that he would fall asleep and leave a kettle boiling.

Michael had spent a lot of time preparing the apartment in this manner, since it had been in a shabby condition when he had rented it. Two friends, Lynda and Ryan, with whom he had studied architecture, had rented the apartment for him. They realized that he would require accommodation upon his return from teaching for a privileged language school for executives in Kobe, Japan. A police SWAT team had taken the previous drug-dealing tenant into custody, and when the apartment became available Lynda and Ryan had applied for it in Michael's name. Hard work and careful planning had made it very hospitable. He had lived in it four years, so far. Until the past year, he had been healthy and happy.

My mind mulled over that afternoon when Michael had explained to me that he was gay. I had taken a year's leave of absence from teaching that year, and was completing my course work and proposal for my doctoral degree. Michael had been studying his professional degree in architecture at Waterloo University then, and we had been able to share some week-ends in Toronto. Often we would spend the time together at the Robarts Library, searching through stacks of books to complete assignments. It was fun being with him, and I was delighted whenever he called and requested breakfast...and the use of my library card.

One sunny, but cold, winter afternoon we were walking up Yonge Street towards the St. George graduate residence where I lived, when he stopped at a leather store.

"That's just what I need, Mom. A pair of black leather pants."
"Oh, Michael. You don't need them! They'll think that you're gay. How about some new jeans instead?"
He looked at me very steadily, and said, "No, I have all the jeans that I need."

We kept walking, but once we were back at the residence, he sat beside me on my bed and said, "Mom, I need to talk to you." I

NOT A TOTAL WASTE

wondered what was wrong. His architectural courses were intensely demanding, so that I assumed his concerns were study-related. I put down the documents that I had been showing him, and waited.

"Mom, remember the leather pants discussion?"
"Yes. Mike, if you really want them, we can go back and get them. I could use some of my scholarship money. They could be an early birthday present!"
"No, that's not it, Mom. I have to let you know this. I AM GAY, and you need to understand that."
I looked at him, and quickly reached for his hand. "Oh, Michael. I didn't mean to hurt you. I'm sorry".
"Sorry...that I'm gay?" His face seemed pinched and tight. His eyes watched me warily.
"No, Mike. No. In case I might have hurt your feelings. It's no big deal to me if you are gay. I love you. I'll always love you-- no matter what. It just doesn't matter."

We looked at each other steadily, through our eyes and into our souls. Simultaneously, we reached for each other, hugged tightly and kissed cheeks.

"But please promise to take care of yourself, dear, because I'm honestly afraid. I've read about gay bashings by gangs in The Star last week. They act like a pack of blood-thirsty hyenas. There are a lot of crazy people out there who would hurt you. Look at what is happening with the recent raids on the baths. Even the police seem to have acted with ignorance and brutality."
"I know that Mom. I am careful. But it was important to me that I let you know."

I reached out and pulled Michael towards me, not wanting to let him leave. I yearned to shield him against the world's hysteria-- to protect him from any slight. It was not necessary to search too hard for blatant examples of our society's discriminatory and irrational policies. Perhaps he had anticipated my need to shelter him. He smiled, as he gently patted my shoulder. In a softened voice, he explained that he had promised to meet Travis and some friends for supper before heading back to university.

I watched him from my window as he entered the courtyard below. He raised his head, smiled, waved cavalierly, and was gone. Oh Michael, my only precious son. What pain you've been carrying alone, these many years. Now I could comprehend some of his self-imposed isolation while he went through high school. Some of the bullying which he had tolerated, and his loneliness were probably not only related to his studious, gentle nature. Perhaps his personal sexual preferences had been obvious to classmates. He'd had both male and female friendships, but I couldn't recall his dating much until his senior year. Sherry had been a special friend, missed by the entire family after her return to New Zealand. They still kept in touch, but she was a wife and mother now. He had often seemed so forlorn, depressed and uncommunicative. Many hours had been spent sequestered in his room, reading. Mike had seldom taken part in extra-curricular activities.

I felt inadequate, distressed that I could not have saved him from some of that pain. Even now, any effort on my part would be futile. I was helpless. I kept thinking of the number of young men brutalized by red-neck fools, who would blatantly destroy anything that they could not comprehend. My stomach became cramped when I thought of the self-righteous bible-thumpers. Those homophobics would point fingers in disapproval, rather than offer an open hand in friendship and love. Surely God is love--not condemnation--to all of us.

I must have studied two dozen books in the next few days, obsessively reading everything that I could find to better understand Michael's proclaimed life style. Most of the books came from the Glad Day bookstore on Yonge Street. It seemed that my more academic stores simply didn't cover this topic very thoroughly. Homosexuality was not new to me, but I didn't want my ignorance to offend or upset Michael. I needed to research, to intellectualize my emotions, to grab any bit of data or information that might clarify things for me. Michael was an essential and important part of my life. I was truly grateful that he had felt secure enough to finally come out of the closet. I yearned to provide any support which he might need. In no way did I want our relationship to be threatened by my stupidity. I wanted him to take pride in his many talents, his concern for others, and his altruistic desire to make the world a better place. How can you explain that you love your children nonjudgmentally, forever?

NOT A TOTAL WASTE

Perhaps since I had gained respect for the attributes of so many gay men and lesbian women through my artistic studies, I felt no negative connotations regarding a homosexual life style. I had many homosexual close friends in the visual and literary arts. I didn't fully comprehend what this entailed, sexually, but I was not homophobic. I feared only the rejection, ostracism and pain that society could potentially inflict upon Michael.

Michael was truly a handsome young man, six-foot one-inch in height, weighing 180 lbs., with wavy light golden-blonde hair and clear blue eyes. He wore contacts most days, or sometimes wire-framed "John Lennon" glasses. His favourite clothing seemed to be the softly-washed blue jeans and jacket with white T-shirts, but when he was attired in his good grey suit, shirt, tie and polished shoes he looked very sophisticated. His silk shirts were wildly extravagant. Whenever we went out to dinner, I felt a genuine pride in his demeanour. Sidelong glances from strangers, who must have wondered why this young stud was out with an older woman, made me want to giggle like a school girl. He especially loved it when the waiter saw that I paid the cheque--he said that he felt like a "kept man". His gentle grin and impish, sparkling eyes attracted friends easily, and his loyalty and intelligence retained them. He had been an honour student throughout his education, and Bruce and I had willingly financed his studies throughout the world, as our own splendid Canadian ambassador.

I recalled that before Michael had entered grade nine we ascertained that both he and his older sister, Anna, should undergo vocational inventory testing. We hoped that a determination of their interests and abilities would provide some recommendation towards selecting their school options. Neither of them had any ideas related to future career choices. The testing was a very positive experience. We affirmed that Michael would require constant challenges in order to maintain his interest in school. Anna came in closely behind him in the measurement and evaluation process so that we held high expectations for her, too. Our only concern was related to the liver problems which she had battled. We hoped that her physical strength would not be a deterrent for her future studies.

Because Michael had been blessed with a brilliant mind, we decided to hold the carrot of "possible world travel" in front of him. He took his first school trip to France in grade nine, one to Italy in grade ten, visited the Canary Islands in grade eleven, studied for a year in Brazil as an exchange student, and then concentrated on his grade thirteen courses to ensure his chance for scholarships. His linguistic skills rapidly expanded. During university Michael studied in Rome for a year, Paris for two years, England for half a year, and toured Europe a few times. He acquired proficiency in six languages, and comprehended three others.

In the last year of his architectural degree studies, Michael dealt with a few tragedies which profoundly affected him. The first was the loss of his best friend, James, who was killed by a drunk driver. James had been the brother that Michael had always wanted. Michael had been best man at James' and Betty's wedding and godfather to their daughter. He loved them all very much, and losing James was a bitter blow. He maintained contact with Betty and Samantha, and visited frequently, until his own death. Betty was never told that his last long bicycle ride on his "Green Mountain Rider" was out to the Beaches, to say his farewell. He had not called Betty, but had intended to surprise her and Samantha. They were not home when he arrived, and he was truly exhausted by the time he returned to his apartment.

A few months after James' death, just prior to the Christmas holiday, Michael called home. His voice sounded extremely upset. One of the young men in the apartment had called his folks to let them know he'd be late for the holiday. He had make-up-work to complete on one of his courses. The architecture degree is not an easy one, and he had failed one course. Additional work was required during his vacation, in order to remain in the program. The young man's father became hostile and told him not to bother coming home for the season at all, and hung up on him.

The stress from overstudying and parental disapproval was too much for the young man, and he committed suicide. Michael had found his body, and phoned me. Coming so soon after losing James, this second death impacted strongly upon Michael. His decision to spend the holiday with Stephan in Toronto, seemed wise. I had urged him to come home, but he needed some space and time to heal. Two weeks later, he seemed calm and composed after that brief vacation, when he called me. He was determined to persist with his studies.

NOT A TOTAL WASTE

Three months later, his last room-mate suffered an epileptic seizure while showering and drowned. Michael had tried to resuscitate him, but to no avail. The anxiety and pathos which came across in his telephone call to me, still reverberate in my mind. After we talked, he hastily packed and vacated the apartment. He had nervously chirped, "I'm out of here, Mom." That week-end, Michael moved into Stephan's apartment in Toronto.

Despite the fact that he was so close to completion of his Master's degree in architecture, he decided not to return to those studies. Memories were too raw and painful for him and he was at loose ends for six months. He worked as a waiter in Toronto and slowly got his life together. I visited him one week-end and we discussed what he might do to get back on track. He couldn't seem to think of any specific study route at the time, so his father and I offered him funding to go to Paris and immerse himself in the French language for a year. He loved that experience. His pronunciation and syntax were superlative upon his return and he seemed more at ease.

After supporting himself as a waiter that summer, Michael left for Japan to teach English to executives at Kobe. He wrote beautiful, frequent letters during that year. One of these was in response to our query about his future career prospects. His father and I had recommended that he return home, take a Master of Arts degree and perhaps an English as a Second Language course. Although a pre-test might have been required, we had not anticipated that it would have posed him any problem. I'd like to share his letter with you.

Dear Ma,

Thanks for all the letters and all the help. I greatly appreciate it. However, I have decided to become a fireman. JOKE!

I have decided to come home, for the very simple reason that it will be much easier for me to do the things I need to do at home, and then IF I get accepted for my Masters I will need to be settled. I may also need to write a language entrance exam for the English as a Second Language studies, and will need a chance to study. Besides that, a complete lunatic has moved into the house (a serious lunatic!) and my tolerance for Japan and being a racial minority has gone right out the window. I also want to check into a lot of possiblities (i.e. Woodsworth, University of Waterloo, etc...). Did I say "simple reason"? I am also homesick, and the job is not nearly as profitable as I had hoped. Living here is EXPENSIVE, and saving has become quite difficult. My living expenses are around $1,000/month, and I am NOT being extravagant. I go out maybe twice a month.

I saw "Out of Africa" the other day. It was a good movie. I enjoyed it. The only other movie I have gone to here is "Blade Runner". A movie costs $12.00 and there is no crowd control, so you have to fight your way through the people coming out to get a seat, and they always sell more tickets than seats (about 20% more). A movie here is not usually a pleasant experience. Out of Africa was. I never was crazy about Meryl Streep before, but this time she was AMAZING (even if she did use the Danish accent when she should have been speaking Danish to her husband).

I am sitting in my Tanaka class now (the bust of Mr. Tanaka is glowering down at me as I write this) but I am alone. Miss Kayama is leaving the company, so her friends have gone to say goodbye to her (i.e. my students) and there will be none of them here except maybe Mr. Yamamoto, later. This means we will be discussing the finer points of his "Proposal for Energy Formation in the Sewage Sludge Incinerator System". Does that sound like fun or does that sound like fun? I get PAID to do this. Isn't life strange?

Congratulations once again, on your Supervisory Officer's Papers. I understand how much all that returned free time must mean to you. Et le francais, comment ca va? Moi, j'en ai tout oublie. Je crois qu'il faut encore un an a Paris apres l'ecole pour que je poisse en apprendre. Ca veut dire, apres un M.A.

I am not sure, exactly how this M.A. thing works. Can I TEACH after it, or do I have to get a teaching degree? I don't understand...could I go to Paris and get my degree in French from the Sorbonne, and then teach French with the M.A.? I am tres confused. What are my chances of getting in? I asked for the two professors that you mentioned--was that a good choice?

LATER--I just found this letter. I had better send it now or you may never get it. Hope you are well--say hi to everyone for me. Love, Michael.

NOT A TOTAL WASTE

I remember sitting in Bemelmans' restaurant on Bloor Street that beautiful day in late June 1986, after Michael's return from Japan. He appeared tired and solemn.

"Mike, what's wrong? Is it just the exhaustion of the trip?"
"No, Ma, I just don't know what I'm going to do now. I get depressed every time I have to make decisions about my future."

"Oh, well--let's look at these, then."

I spread seven acceptance letters across the table for him to look at, from various universities. While he had been in Japan, I had sent applications with his transcripts to several different universities, for a few programs that my husband and I had hoped Michael might consider for his future. We knew that he had to complete his education in order to be gainfully employed, and certainly did not want him to spend the rest of his life wondering about a potential career change.

"What's this, Mom?"
"Read them, and decide which one you would prefer to attend."

I smiled, and watched the excitement grow on his face. The grin and sparkling eyes returned. He looked at me happily and said,

"You're not kidding me? Ontario Institute for Studies in Education has accepted me for a Master of Arts degree. My B.Sc. marks were acceptable? Did they include the marks from my Master's in Architectural studies? Can I actually go?"
"Yes. Dad and I will cover the costs. Once you earn your Master's degree, you should have no problem getting into Teacher's College, or else you could pursue your Doctoral degree. Your letter did mention returning to Paris to continue French courses. That's a viable alternative after getting the Masters. You decide! We know that you'll do fine, Michael. We just want you to be happy, and to finish your education. What do you think?"

He was joyous, exuberant, thrilled. I had been a bit nervous that he might have resented my pre-planning his life for him upon his return from Japan. I was relieved that he felt this jubilant. I still feel warm and happy when I remember seeing him sitting there, not quite believing his luck. He had the tools to move ahead with his life, now.

Michael completed his Master's degree courses with his usual high honours and then did the same thing with Teacher's College. He had left the Master's thesis undone, but had made a good start at it, and intended to complete it later. In September of 1989, he started to teach elementary school.

By November of that year the Axidothymidine (AZT) medication had stopped working and his health had begun to quickly deteriorate. Despite the realization that this had been a possibility, I felt a mounting panic. Little was known then about the high toxicity of the drug AZT. Some infected people now refer to it as AIDS in the bottle, because some people react poorly to its use. Studies are still being done on its real value. When Mike had lived with Stephan, he had explained to me that Stephan had AIDS-related complex, a precursor to full-blown AIDS. He had called it ARC, which was actually an early stage of AIDS. Stephan had severe weight loss, swollen lymph nodes, fever, fatigue, chronic diarrhea and frequent flu-like illnesses. I had known Stephan for a few years and grown fond of him. His decline was viewed with alarm.

Stephan's friends generously compensated for his initial lack of parental support. The lack of familial involvement in many AIDS-related illnesses amazed me, but I learned that this ostracism also occurred because the patient refused reliance upon relatives who had previously acted in a punative manner. In some cases, they also wished their illness to be kept secret, so that it would not impact upon their families in any way. It seemed that Stephan had stubbornly determined not to notify his family regarding his illness, but during that last month they were located in Florida and informed by his friends. Although his father had still spurned him, his mother immediately flew to his side. She remained with him until his death, shared Stephan's time and offered supplemental help. In one way, Stephan was more fortunate than many AIDS patients. He did not die as a lonely, societal castoff and a victim of self-destruction. Near the end of Stephan's life, Michael would not permit me to attend their weekly visits. He carried the flowers, groceries and records to him, alone. All that I could do was to write and send hand-knitted socks to keep Stephan's toes warm.

NOT A TOTAL WASTE

When Stephan died of pneumocystis carinii pneumonia, Michael had calmly explained to me that he also had tested positively for antibodies to the HIV virus. This was the virus thought to cause the "opportunistic" infection which had killed Stephan. The AIDS-related illness, or Acquired Immunodeficiency Syndrome had collapsed Stephan's immune system. I had stared at Michael in disbelief when he told me about Stephan and cried without shame when he confirmed his own infection. I expressed anger that AIDS had been rejected by researchers because it was initially considered to be a homosexual disease. The number of deaths from AIDS would continue to skyrocket throughout the world. We discussed its wanton destruction for hours during that interminable night. In an effort to appease me, Michael had explained that someone who is HIV positive might not develop full-blown AIDS for a decade. Although nothing was known for certain about AIDS, Michael felt confident that he would not get sick for anywhere from eight to twelve years. We had walked and talked for what seemed like hours that night. We both wept. I remember asking him if he and Stephan had been lovers, and he said that they had only been friends and "roomies". They had lived in the same apartment and known many mutual friends, but they had not been lovers.

With the onset of AIDS, Michael had resigned, and left behind the chosen career he had loved so much. He had proven that he was a natural teacher, and his students valued him. His ability to reach each of his English As A Second Language students through their own language, endeared him to immigrant youngsters who felt alien in a strange country. The extra time that he took to contact parents when the students had difficulty in their Mathematics or Science classes, and to prepare individual enrichment materials helped each student to blossom. His own artistic creativity was shared in his Art and Drama classes, encouraging the students to achieve their best potential. His sense of wit and dry humour turned many an awkward classroom situation around, and the students responded with affection. Michael's sense of fair but firm discipline taught the students to respect authority. His friendliness to the students gave them confidence to share personal worries and anxieties, and obtain his intensive listening. He was a fine teacher, and he had worked hard to achieve this career. Leaving it behind was truly a distressing time for him, and for us.

His doctor now urged him to take a part-time sedentary occupation, to provide structure in his life. For awhile, Mike worked selling theatre tickets through telephone solicitation, and computerized transactions. This also allowed him to remain financially independent as long as possible. This was an important element of Michael's self-esteem. When the physical demands of that job became too difficult, his insurance assisted him to cover his debts.

This erosion of his health was not obvious in his attitude towards life. Michael was optimistic and cheerful in his goals for the future. I do not remember him complaining about health weaknesses, nor did he ever make derogatory comments about anyone. Whenever I did, he turned his famous scowl upon me, lifted his eyebrows, and waited for me to apologize. He would not continue the conversation until I had played his "Synectics" game and provided a few positive observations for the person in question. I often felt uncomfortable, trying to be that noble. He would grin at me and chide me for my criticism. He remained loving, and concerned for others.

CHAPTER THREE

All of those thoughts had marched progressively through my mind as I sat waiting for Michael to shower. Once he was dressed, we wasted little time in ordering a taxi. We arrived at the hospital Admitting Department by noon, and waited for over an hour before we were moved to a second waiting area. The trip preparations and sitting in the wheel chair for an hour had left Michael exhausted; he promptly fell asleep on the gurney behind the curtained cubicle. I remained beside him throughout that afternoon. By eight o'clock that night, after he had been probed and checked by four doctors, I felt a mounting hysteria. Michael's breathing had become shallow, his colour was ashen, and he twitched and trembled as if he could have an epileptic seizure. The palpable frustration which I felt from witnessing his steady decline, forced me to act.

I left him alone for a few moments to locate the young intern that had signed us into the hospital. As he rushed past me in the hall, I begged him for an intravenous feeding for Michael immediately. He stared at me, and I blurted out,

"Look, for God's sake, Michael has been here since noon and has not had any fluids. He's shaking as if he's going to have a seizure, and no-one will help me. He must have fluids right away!"

The doctor stepped back and stared at me, and then said, "Of course, you're right. I've got the IV person just around the corner. Go back to your son, and I'll get the IV started right away."

Why had it taken over eight hours to have Michael admitted to a private room? Why was everything tortuously slow? It seemed barbarous to force us both to painfully wait and wait. Once the intravenous was started, his colour began to improve. Within half an hour a colleague of Dr. Baker, the doctor we had originally expected to have admitted Michael, appeared beside his bed. She explained that Michael was scheduled to have a CAT scan, followed by a spinal tap. Apparently, Dr. Baker would not be seeing him until the following morning, once all of the test results were available.

The doctor then asked more of the identical questions which Michael had been answering all afternoon. He kept his eyes shut now, and took his time in responding. We waited for his soft, thoughtful replies. Slowly, he would complete the sentences with the required words. This city was...Toronto. He was in...an unknown hospital. His name was Michael. The day of the week was...not known. He was thirty-two years of age. The year was...unknown. The last country that he had visited in was...France. He was painfully slow in this process, which alarmed me. What was holding him back? Why was he so reticent before he completed each statement? Why was he having difficulty with some of the answers? The doctor appeared to be rushed, and after a curt, "Fine, Michael", she turned on her heel and left the cubicle.

Shortly after her departure, things seemed to speed up. Before I realized it, Michael was in a hospital gown, IV hooked up, diapers in place, and they were wheeling him down the hall for the CAT scan. I stood beside his bed watching him leave. I felt like shouting for them not to take him away. Fear tugged at my heart. I was terrified that I would never see him again. He looked up at me, grinned and winked. Then, he was gone.

"You'll have to leave now, Maria. This usually takes a few hours, and he will not be able to see you once he has had the spinal tap. Get some rest, and come back in the morning," advised the doctor.

Even though I didn't want to leave, I realized that the tension of the day had weighed heavily upon me. My eyes burned with fatigue, and my shoulders felt as tight as steel bands. My lower back throbbed, and my middle-aged feet were swollen to twice their size. The joints of my jaw were so tensed that I wondered if they would click if I tried to speak. Slowly, I realized that it was necessary to get some rest, in order to deal with the next morning. I located a telephone in the lobby, and called home to my husband. After giving Bruce what little information I had to offer, he assured me that he and the grandchildren were fine. He said that they could cope without me as long as it was necessary, and to concentrate on giving Michael whatever assistance he needed. My husband's emotional support provided some relief, yet my heart felt very heavy as I started back to the apartment.

Penny met me in the kitchen when I got back, and greeted me with,

"Well, is he dead?"

I froze in the middle of the room, and struggled to respond. "No, I don't think so."

"Oh, well if he is, then I want the kettle, the computer, the stereo..."

This attempt at wry humour was more than I could handle. Tears stung my eyes, and I stumbled towards the dining room futon. Nothing came to my mind in response and I lay down with my back to Penny. I tried to control the tears that wanted to flood the room. Pessimism dampened my hopes for Michael's recovery from this horrendous viral disease. I could no longer fool myself. No cure had been found for any other known virus. No immunity had been developed for previous viral infections. The world seemed to remain oblivious to the real dangers of AIDS.

She went to the kitchen and came back with a small glass of Irish Cream liqueur. I shook my head and turned away, but her hand came forward firmly.

"Take it, Maria. You must slow down and sleep. Michael will need you to be strong for him tomorrow. Call me at the office if you need anything. By the way, if Mike needs a blood transfusion, please tell them that I am willing to help out."

I sipped the drink without feeling any more relaxed. Gradually exhaustion overcame me, and I tried to doze off. In retrospect, Penny had not realized that my tension and terror over Michael's illness mentally blocked out her attempt to help me. I was well aware of her good friendship with Michael. However, at that time I could not comprehend her humour, and wanted only to be held, like a child, while I wept. It was too soon for me to be strong and brave. My vulnerability overruled logic, which was unusual for me. She was sickened at the prospect of losing a dear friend. I was in shock that I would lose my only son. I made a concentrated effort to slow down. I breathed more deeply and attempted to organize my thoughts. The city street sounds came through the window, exaggerated by my tension. I awoke with a start each time I heard a noise, and then sunk into a fitful slumber. I heard Penny leave for work after eight, and then the phone rang shortly after nine.

It was Michael's friend, David. We chatted briefly, and I gave him what information I had on Michael's condition. He promised to be at the hospital that evening--and he kept that commitment almost each night that Michael was hospitalized. He would arrive an hour before visiting hours were ended, to chat with both of us. Afterwards, he would insist on driving me back to the centre of the city to Michael's apartment.

Along the way, he always encouraged me to try to eat supper, despite the late hour. How he located such beautiful patio restaurants all over the city, I'll never know. I did try to taste soups and eat some solids, but stress developed a large blockage in my throat. This imaginary growth prevented any food passage. This same apprehension over Michael's declining health removed flavours and smells from food. The best meals tasted flat, devoid of seasoning. Trying to swallow caused gagging. This malady would recur frequently, from that summer and long past Michael's death. I was probably the most reluctant dinner guest that David had ever entertained. David was both patient and persistent. He provided daily encouragement that helped to strengthen me throughout that long, hot summer.

NOT A TOTAL WASTE

Six months after Michael's death, Kim detailed how deeply David's own pain had affected him during that exhausting, frightening time. All the while that David had guaranteed that I took some sustenance, he suffered his own lack of appetite. David graciously drove me home after my hospital visits with Michael, and wished me a good rest. Kim spent many nights calming David afterwards, and encouraging him to seek quiet repose.

Both Ted and Corey showed their concern for Michael, and called and visited him on a regular basis. They seemed to take turns in helping him to eat his meals. When he was too weak to feed himself, they spoonfed him. Michael would try harder to eat for them, and I would just relax and watch. He was determined not to give up when he had this much love offered. Penny, Lucy and Therese also visited sporadically. Gradually, he tolerated the curtains being opened; as the fever was reduced, his eyes became less sensitive to the sunlight.

CHAPTER FOUR

On the third day Dr. Baker came in to check on him while I was seated beside his bed, reading. She introduced herself to me and then invited me to come down the hall. It had been a source of irritation to me that most of the doctors and interns rarely addressed Michael directly. They asked me how Michael felt, and discussed treatment as though he were invisible. It seemed a cruelty that was based upon ignorance. This had occurred while Corey visited. Finally, he erupted with,

"Why don't you ask Mike? He's conscious. Look, he's right there!"

I felt the same frustration at this time, but was afraid to upset Michael, or to incur the doctor's resentment. It amazed me that the medical staff, in general, seemed intent on dehumanizing the patient by stripping him of all feelings of hope, or control over his own situation. My eyes met Michael's, and he turned his face towards the wall. Obediently, I followed Dr. Baker out of the room.

"You know why I asked you to come down this way, don't you?"

"I guess it's so that Michael cannot hear your diagnosis. What is wrong?"

"You know what he has, don't you? You know why he is sick?"

"I thought that you would tell me."
"He has full-blown AIDS. Didn't you realize he was HIV positive before this?"
"Yes. But what is it that is causing the related infections?"
"We did a CAT scan, some additional X-rays and a spinal tap. We've drawn blood, stool and urine samples."
"Yes, I'm well aware of that. And the results?"
"We've found lesions in his brain, in his bowel, lungs, and throat. The lesions in the brain and abdomen are the biggest concerns right now."
"What does this mean?"
"With cancerous lesions in his brain, he has maybe two weeks or less, at a maximum of eight weeks."
"No, I can't believe this. Can cancerous lesions grow that quickly? He was fine two weeks ago, just thin and tired. I just can't believe this."
"Well, face it. It happens."
"Wait. I believe he has an infection--something that a strong antibiotic can help. Why can't you check on that?"
"Look, I've given you the diagnosis. Accept it. He's going to need you to be strong and supportive."
"But I want some more testing done. This diagnosis must be incorrect. This is Michael's first real illness. He can't have such a short time."
"You knew that he was going to die. The lesions are clearly indicated on the X-rays. Look, this is a terrible disease, but he's not the first one. It's terminal. You can't fight it."

I stood very still, rigid with shock and anger. Slowly she faced me, looked calmly into my eyes and said, "If you have any other family members, this is the time to notify them. I'll be in to see your son, Michael, tomorrow."

She pivoted quickly and darted down the hall, her white lab coat flapping. I wanted to shout, to scream, to chase after her and make her change her diagnosis. I had only empathy for Michael. He had not sought this sickness. My anger was directed squarely at that blunt-mannered doctor, and not at the illness. I felt as though the petite, beautiful, and unfeeling doctor had just squeezed the blood from my veins. My legs couldn't seem to move of their own accord. It was as if they were welded in some manner at the hips, and I had to employ a swinging motion to laboriously move the legs forward.

A trembling began, first slowly, and then more strongly until my body seemed to vibrate of its own accord. I stood against the wall, hugging myself, trying to gain momentum over a bizarre body gone amok. I could not tolerate this dysfunctioning lack of control over myself, nor over Michael's health. I had towered over the doctor, my five foot nine inches against her five feet two, and I had wanted to shake the truth out of her.

How cowardly of her, to leave me to clarify the diagnosis to Michael by myself! How could a health care professional be so remiss in responding to Michael's and my needs? His physical death had not yet occurred. If this was his final act of living, did it not deserve validity? If he was truly incurably ill, why couldn't there be integrity in communicating his prognosis directly to him, and an attitude of support to face this tragedy? While he lived, was there not hope? Why thwart any possible attempt to fight back? How could we break down our anxieties into smaller component parts, to deal with them more effectively? We needed guidance and calm reassurance. We must be permitted to cling to our hopes.

The doctor's callous composure had appeared to emphasize that she had all of the answers. Some intuitive gut-level feeling told me that, as Michael's mother, I knew more than the doctor. Michael and I would prove her to be wrong. We would force ourselves to face our terror of the unknown, loss of Michael's physical and intellectual control, loss of bodily functions, and possible mutilation, decomposition, depression, anger, withdrawal, detachment or sorrow. Our litany of concerns were presently overwhelming. We would pray for the courage to struggle and aspire to increase Michael's life span. I returned to his room in shock and tried hard to appear rational. Michael was in the bathroom. I was grateful, since this allowed me a few moments to pull myself together, before I had to face his questions.

He came out of the bathroom, sat down at a chair facing the mirror and attempted to shave himself. I sat very still and observed him, unable to offer any assistance. He completed those ablutions and then brushed his hair.

"Mom, can you help me to brush my teeth? I can't find the toothpaste, and I want to gargle with some mouthwash to take away the metallic taste that comes from the drugs."

NOT A TOTAL WASTE

I found the items that he needed, and stood behind his chair, facing him in the mirror. My hand rested lightly on his shoulder, needing the solace of his touch. Our eyes met, and he spoke softly,

"I love you, Mom. I'm sorry that you have to go through this with me."

Tears came immediately to my eyes, but I blinked them away.

"Oh, Mike, don't say that. If you only knew...I'm just glad that I'm here. You could have become sick half-way around the world and I wouldn't have been able to help you at all. We'll get through this together, Mike. I love you too, son."

How deeply I loved this young man, and how much I depended upon his joy in life to keep me pushing one foot in front of another. Over the years his dry humour and bright intelligence had been precious gifts, cherished by his friends and loved ones. Mike had truly lived a great deal more during his brief lifetime, than many ever do in twice that many years. I leaned down over the back of his chair and kissed him on his cheek.

He patted my hand, grinned, and gave me a saucy wink in the mirror. I followed his lead, and tried to 'lighten up'. While he stood shakily on his feet, I changed his soiled nightgown and helped him back into his freshly-made bed. In a few moments the nurse arrived and put the catheter roll-on tube in place. He resented having to use that, and he hated the IV, but he leaned back against his pillows and settled down in preparation for sleep. Corey had left classical music and easy-listening tapes with his ghetto-blaster. These played softly as he napped. The CBC classical music was left on during the evenings, and occasionally he would also watch the videos that Corey rented for him. Ted came often at the end of his long day at Lime Ricky's. Where these friends found the stamina to go that "extra mile" each day I'll never know, but their high energy levels and zany humour kept both Michael and me functioning.

Michael had just closed his eyes when Corey came into his room.

"Hi, Maria. How long has Mike been asleep?"
"Oh, Corey, he just closed his eyes. He'll probably wake up in about half an hour, again."

"How about going downstairs to the coffee shop with me?"
"I guess it would be okay, as long as we won't be too long. His doctor was here."
"Come along then, and you can tell me what she gave you as the diagnosis."

We sat at a corner table, sipping the putrid machine made coffee and trying to sort out the medical verdict. The idea of lymphoma, scattered everywhere throughout Michael's body, did not seem feasible. I tried to explain my skepticism to Corey, but choked on the words. He quietly took one of my hands in his, and said,

"You have to be there for Michael. Hang on. He needs you. I know how he feels. You see, I'm HIV positive, too."

I stared into his intelligent, handsome features. Corey was about six foot two, weighed around 185 lbs., had black curly hair and deep brown eyes. He was handsome enough to be a male model, and he loved smart clothes and good parties. Travel took up most of his week-ends; his charm captivated everyone that he met. I couldn't believe that he, too, would be stigmatized by society because of this miserable disease.

"Oh, no, not you too. Do your parents know?"
"No, but they don't know that I'm gay, either. I cannot tell them--ever. They would not be there for me."
"Corey...Oh my God, Corey...there is no way that you should have to handle all of this by yourself. No one should feel that isolated. You can't go through this alone. Corey...then, I will just have to adopt you. Please let me help. You can count on me."

I felt awkward and foolish, trying to explain the impact of emotion that whirled through my mind. How many more of Mike's friends would experience the pathos associated with this disease? Would they obtain the psychological, physical, legal, ethical and economic support which they would need? Medical benefits seemed to be aimed primarily at restoring an individual to a functional health level. Someone battling to survive from day to day was almost shamed into giving up. Logically, hospitals must not waste money on aggressive and costly therapy for a terminally ill patient. Michael did not demand over-treatment, but he did expect quality care to improve his brief remaining life. Terminal illness was expensive, but that did not mean it was less vital.

NOT A TOTAL WASTE

"I won't do a perfect job, Corey. I sure as hell can't cook a fancy meal for you. It's just that...you've been there for my son. You are an important part of his life. Let me be a link between you and Mike. Please promise that when this is all over with Michael, you will keep in touch. I will try to help. Let me be your surrogate mother. Michael would want that."

I choked back the need of a universal wail against this disease that destroyed young lives. AIDS was stealing our children, and no-one seemed to care. How could society virtually ignore this disease? The situation seemed so hopeless. Would it be considered more tragic if it were a unique heterosexual disease? In order to avoid the evolution of an overwhelming experience of death, similar to the plagues of the fourteenth century, the disease must be slowed down.

What means must be employed to make our young, sexually active risk takers fully aware of this potential for calamity? Did they read the advertisements, listen to the prophets, buy condoms, or practice safe sex? AIDS was everyone's problem. No one was immortal. What choices remained? Should specific sexual knowledge be explained to Jenni and Sean, and all other youngsters over the age of eight? Society was generally instructing them about protection against drugs, at that age. Should free condoms and disposable needles be readily available? Was society prepared to provide medical and social costs for an expanding population suffering from reduced functioning and restricted life expectancies, due to AIDS-related illnesses? I doubted that the 'virgin clubs' which were expanding into the secondary schools would be the final answer to this crisis. Monogamous relationships and the refusal of pre-marital sex sounded like great alternatives for stopping the spread of AIDS, but they were not always realistic options for every segment of society.

Corey patted my hand gently, and said, "Come on. I understand what you're trying to say. It will be okay. I'll keep in touch. Promise. First, let's check on Mike, and then it'll be time to get you home. I'll drive you home to-night."

We pushed open the door and were grateful to see that he was not alone. Around Michael's bed stood Lucy, Therese and Ted. Corey and I were amazed that these friends had all arrived so quickly. Flowers now filled the window ledge, and boxes containing tempting date squares, brownies, and Michael's very favourite coconut-cream pie, were on his food table. Bottles of coca-cola and juices were already opened on his bedside tray. Brightly-coloured ribbons ran from one nail to another across the wall which faced Michael. Silver helium balloons and get-well cards hung from these. The curtains were still drawn against the brightness of the sun, which hurt Michael's sensitive eyes. The bed lights gave a cheerful, soft glow. The room appeared festive, and filled with love. Behind Michael was a corkboard, and someone had stapled an enlarged photocopy which Corey had brought. The newspaper print of Roseanne Barr's gesture, made while she sang the national anthem, had created a furor. Seeing it hung there made all of us dissolve into laughter. We badly needed that amusement.

Abstractly, I reached forward and touched Michael's forehead, and realized that it was scalding to the touch. His face was highly flushed.

"Michael, you're awfully hot. Are you feeling worse?"
"Just warm, Mom. Everybody's here, hmm?"
"Yes, they are. But I'm worried about your fever."

At that moment, Michael reached up and pushed at the adjustment dial on his intraveneous feeder. Within a second the drip had increased to a speed that was too rapid. We watched in amazement, and then I turned to Lucy. Her eyes registered the same concern, and she ran to get a nurse. This was very unlike Michael's usual logical actions. Why would he do this? A part of me wanted to say, "Good for you, Mike. Retain whatever control you can over your body and its functions!" The other part of me worried that his actions might have some debilitating effect upon his health. The nurse arrived quickly, and adjusted the dial so that the flow was regulated to a slower, steady drip. Michael studied it quizzically for a few seconds and nonchalantly reached forward and speeded it up.

"Michael, stop that. Don't do that, Mike," said Lucy. He turned his head slowly towards her, as if he had not fully comprehended what had upset her. His hand then disappeared underneath the blankets, he casually removed the catheter cover, stretched back against the pillows and closed his eyes.

"What has he done?"
"I think that he has pulled off the catheter," I replied.
"Oh, Michael. I'll go and get the nurse again."

The nurse asked us to leave while she made him clean and comfortable, since the bedclothes and his nightgown would require changing. Michael detested depending upon a catheter, and consistently removed this, leaving a messy bed as a result. This defiant stance was abnormal behaviour for Michael, but then, these were not normal times. I was scared when I noticed the change in his appearance. His eyes were not focusing properly, and his body had become more flushed. He refrained from responding to questions and he kept his eyes shut when we returned. He seemed in a state of limbo, as though he were completely alone in the room. Oblivious to the chatter of his friends, he lay still. The nurse returned and took his temperature, which registered on the computerized thermometer at 104.9 degrees, and I froze in a state of panic. His temperature was dangerously high, and could lead to convulsions, or a stroke.

Outside the door we overheard the Nursing Assistant speaking to the nurse, as she cleared away the soiled bedding.

"Those guys get really high fevers before they die, don't they? They sweat like pigs and use up all the bedding. I had some experience in my country with them. You got to be careful how you clean them up. You can catch it from them, if you're not. They just wet, shit and puke."

The nurse responded coldly, "He has a high fever, but we'll bring it down."

My cheeks burned with anger over the ignorance of that particular Nursing Assistant. Still, Michael's fever was a more legitimate concern. It didn't seem to be getting lower. Within an hour I went to the nurse's station and asked if they were going to give him any additional medication to bring it back to normal. They said that they were waiting for a doctor to see him, and could not give medication without authority. I asked if there were any other doctors nearby, and recalled the young intern who had helped me in the admitting room. He had said that I could have him paged at any time and given me the hours when he was on duty. I asked the nurse to call him for me and she promised to do that later. I did not believe that she would call for him, but just intended to soothe me. Her flippant manner gave me no boost in confidence. I felt subservient, frightened and angry. Mike should not be treated as if he was both socially and physically dead already. My trust quotient was very low.

I returned to Michael's room, but could not keep the tears from stinging my eyes. His friends were solemn, not knowing how to help. After a few moments, my frustration got the best of me. I suddenly grabbed a bottle of rubbing alcohol from his bedside table, wet four facecloths from the bathroom, poured rubbing alcohol onto them, and started to bathe his body from the head down. He didn't move, but groaned softly. I left one cloth wrapped around his chin and onto his cheeks, one on the back of his neck, and one on his forehead. Then, I commenced to cool down the rest of his fragile body. I simply forgot that his friends were there--and concentrated upon beating the fever down. I lost track of time, but I am sure that this continued for two to three hours. Time melted away. When I stretched my stiffened back and looked up, David had somehow displaced all of the others. Our eyes met.

"Maria, the fever is down now, and Michael's still asleep. You can't do any more. It's after ten o'clock. Come with me and get something to eat. You haven't had anything all day, have you?"

"I can't leave him, David. I'm not hungry. I had coffee and muffins earlier. He's not asleep. Look at him; he's unconscious."

"Come on, sweetie. You can't fix it. The nurse said that they'll be giving him some medication soon. You have to leave with me. You can come back in the morning."

I looked at Michael, and knew that David was right. Yet, it tore me to pieces to leave him looking so drawn and helpless. My own exhaustion took its toll, and I started to sob without control. David came close and put his arm around my shoulder, and handed me a freshly-ironed linen hankerchief. I waved it away because I didn't want to mess it up, but David pushed it forward again, saying,

"Nonsense. These are magic. They clear up tears right away, and repair damaged makeup upon contact".

NOT A TOTAL WASTE

I laughed through my tears, and accepted his gallantry. I tiptoed over and kissed Michael's cheek. Then, I let David lead me out of the room, towards the elevators.

As we walked down the hall, David said, "Maria, Kim has borrowed my key to Michael's apartment today. He and his commercial cleaning staff have created a surprise for you. I want you to try to eat something, and then I want to take you home to show you. Also, Penny has left for Edmonton for a few weeks to visit her sister. You'll sleep better, having your privacy. Kim has worked so hard to clean up the apartment for you and for Michael."

We stopped at another enchanting patio restaurant on the way home. The towering trees reached upwards, disappearing into the night sky. David selected a corner table, privately snuggled up against the largest elm. The scent from the summer flowers were wafted by playful breezes, while a string quartet played David's favourite Mozart to enhance the setting. Coloured lights winked playfully, disguising the high, boarded fence which enclosed the eating area. For a brief time, it seemed as though we were in an oasis, far from the stark terror of Mike's illness.

David was patient with my lack of appetite and as he sipped his martini, discussed the music. The quartet played Mozart's last three string quartets, the so-called "Prussian" ones, K. 575, 589 and 590. David explained that those were the ones which Mozart had written to secure a regular court appointment, and were written in 1789-90 when Mozart travelled to Berlin. They were dedicated to an illustrious cellist, King Frederick William II of Prussia, who vainly prided himself in having studied under Duport. Apparently for that reason, the cello was quite prominent in nearly all the movements, but in the middle parts retreated into the background. The reality of the day seemed nearly obliterated, replaced by the expressiveness of the music.

Within an hour, David seemed eager to show me the changes made at the apartment. Upon arrival at Michael's apartment, a fresh clean smell greeted us. Corey had returned Michael's white drapes from the drycleaners, and these were rehung. David had replaced the stained mattress on Michael's bed, and a new exquisitely-designed dark cerulean blue, deep burgundy and silver grey duvet, sheet and pillow sham set made his bedroom look very elegant.

Next to the six foot high window, the rest of the wall was insulated with Mike's beloved mystery and classic books. His clock radio and telephone remained within hand's reach. Opposite the bed was the colour television which David had installed for Michael, and Michael's VCR. Next to the doorway was a three-drawer chest, now scrubbed and devoid of any clutter. Over the bed hung a large ROBOCOP poster (Michael's favourite film), but at eye-level, immediately above the television, David had placed a romantic print of a Parisian street scene.

A Spanish watercolour of Don Quixote, astride his horse and prepared to fight windmills, was located above the dresser. Michael and I frequently chuckled over that one. Cervantes' romantic hero had tried in an extravagantly chivalrous, but unrealistic way, to rescue the oppressed and fight evil during at least eight more adventures after his war with the windmills. He was a model for Michael, who would fight his own windmill attack. The Binimi sculpture of his knight-errant had been a fun gift from me, and he kept this on his book shelf.

The entire apartment had been polished and cleaned by Kim and his staff. The smell of diarrhea had finally been squelched. In its place was a mingling of flowers and disinfectant that was not at all unpleasant. There was no way to express my gratitude properly.

"Now, get some rest so that you'll be ready for Michael tomorrow, Maria. I'll call you in the morning."
"David, thank you--and please thank Kim--and everyone else."
"No problem, sweetie. You just get some rest."

He was gone too quickly for me to hug him. David had illustrated for me the strength and kindness which Mike had valued in their friendship, despite David's own anxiety. My appreciation for his and Kim's help seemed inadequate. Once he was gone, the apartment seemed a desolate place. Mike was not here, and neither was the support and companionship of his many friends. I was very much alone.

CHAPTER FIVE

The next morning, Dr. Baker was already in Michael's room when I arrived. I opened the door to her voice.

"There's no other route, Michael. We must use this invasive technique to determine how extensively the lymphoma is scattered throughout the brain. Once we've determined that, we can assess further treatment. I'll send the neurosurgeon to see you today. You must sign the release papers permitting the brain biopsy."

I stood stock still and scarcely breathed. Michael replied,

"I don't want the surgery. THERE IS NO NEED."
"I'm not here to argue with you, Michael. You want to get well, don't you?"
"Yes, if that's possible. But I refuse any unnecessary treatment."
"What are you telling me?"
"Take a look at my chart. My Mom can explain it to you."

She looked past Michael and gave me a piercing look. I took an automatic step backwards against the wall. Swiftly, she left the room.

David had prepared Michael's Living Will, a Power of Attorney, and his final Will. These had been signed, and copies had been left with his chart at the nursing station. It was at Michael's request that these things had been looked after so swiftly, but a part of me tensed up just considering their full implications. I avoided facing the fact that they might be necessary now, at this time. My heart told me that Michael was going to live forever. Death had to be a long, long way from the present reality.

David had expected me to sleep in Michael's freshly-attired bedroom on the previous night, but I had found that impossible. To my way of thinking, any other use except Michael's would have defiled it, or negated any potential for him to recover. I wanted the apartment to be left unscathed, in preparation for his return from the hospital. I had slept soundly, however, on the dining room futon. If there had been any domestic squabbles in the nearby sprawling apartment complex, I did not hear them. If the mentally-deranged woman down the street had screamed her nightly obscenities to the moon from her balcony, I didn't recall. If there were drunken arguments between the street people as they sojourned to and from the brewery store on the corner, I was unaware. Police, ambulance and cat mating sirens went unheard. I slept without dreams or nightmares, and awoke refreshed and ready to tackle a new day.

As I walked towards the subway on that beautiful July morning, the world acquired a new clarity. The grass peeking between the concrete cracks seemed greener. Flowers nodded from window sills and the city appeared to be disguised in a fresh, new coat of paint. Sparrows chirped over the traffic. It felt good to be alive. Confidence that Michael's health would surely improve with each day, provided an extra spring to my step. Although that brief visit from Dr. Baker had left me feeling uneasy, I clung tightly to every optimistic thought.

By ten o'clock that morning a dark-haired, chunky-set neurosurgeon entered the room with his clipboard and pen poised. In a soft-spoken voice, he queried,

"Michael?"
"Yes.
He introduced himself, and began. "I've been asked to schedule your surgery, tentatively for tomorrow."
"Tomorrow? That decision was not approved when Dr. Baker was here earlier," I said.

NOT A TOTAL WASTE 41

He raised his head from the clipboard, nodded at me and asked, "Are you Michael's mother?"

"That's right. But Michael has made no decision regarding any surgery."

Michael sighed, "I don't want the surgery, Mom. I told Dr. Baker that there is no need."

"Is this a common operation? What are the side effects? Any dangers? What does it accomplish? Why does she want this done?" I threw questions at him like a robot. My fear was only lightly masked behind my urgent need to know his answers.

The surgeon put the clipboard down on Michael's bed and placed his hands on the back of a nearby chair.

"Well, basically the biopsy will provide information required to treat you, Michael." He had turned away from me, and spoke directly to Michael. This allowed me to relax a bit, grateful that he did not expect me to make any final decision. "What does it entail? How do they do it? First of all, we should discuss the negative possibilities. If anything goes wrong, you could suffer a hemorrhage and paralysis from a stroke. You could lose your sight, or impair motor co-ordination. You could also die. Now, if nothing goes wrong, we'll have tissue which can indicate what medication routes we must follow towards your treatment. Should the lesion prove cancerous, then we must make you as comfortable as possible. If it is healthy tissue, then we must test for viral or bacterial presence."

"Is this done routinely?"

"No, Michael. In fact, we try to avoid invasive techniques like this because of the risk factor. Dr. Baker wants to move aggressively to locate the problem and feels that time is a vital element."

"What do we do? Sign a release form?"

"Yes, that's common policy. What's your decision, Michael?"

Michael looked up at the ceiling, sighed and closed his eyes. The doctor and I stood and watched him for a few moments. Mike opened his eyes and looked directly at the doctor, and replied,

"I'll sign it. Mom, we'll give it a try."

"You will both have to sign this."

We did sign, but I felt insecure about the prospect of Michael's surgery. Why hadn't we discussed his decision? He had looked so wan and dejected while he signed that consent form. Should we have had more input, or a second opinion first? Now, Mike appeared resolved that his was the right response. He turned from me, and slept peacefully. This was his judgment. If he wished to proceed, then I would support his wishes.

The next morning I arrived at eight o'clock, because I realized that the assistant neurosurgeon would prepare Michael for the operation, sometime after ten. I wanted to share the interim waiting period with Michael. After picking up coffee and a muffin in the cafeteria, I climbed the flights of stairs to his room in floor G5, the AIDS ward.

His bed was empty. Panic jumped at me from the four corners of that little room. The desk nurse answered with, "Perhaps he's in the sun room, down the hall, or maybe he went for a walk." In disbelief, I ran and checked. He was nowhere to be found. She rechecked the X-ray and surgery schedules for me, and his name was not there. Slowly, I returned to his room and sat beside his bed to wait. I shoved the styrofoam cup and muffin aside, and tried to rationalize. The room was a cold, dreary place, devoid of Michael's personality. CBC classical music played softly in the darkened room. In consideration for Michael's eyesight sensitivity, I did not open the drapes. I sat rigidly, in a state of shock.

An hour later, the young intern who had admitted Michael walked through the doorway, smiled and asked,

"Hi, how's your son doing?"
"I don't know. He's gone."
"Gone?"
"I've been waiting here for nearly two hours. No-one will tell me where he has gone."

He looked at me blankly, and sat down on the stool next to me. My tears came of their own volition. They'd been stemmed for so long, but now my fears were obvious.

"I'm sure that he's all right. I'll go check on it, and come right back."

He patted my arm, and moved quickly away. Within five minutes he returned, with a smile on his face.

NOT A TOTAL WASTE — 43

"Michael is downstairs having a CAT scan and additional X-rays. They are doing essential blood work before he comes up. Somehow this was omitted from his chart. Shall I sit with you awhile?"

"Please. Thank you for locating him. I went a little bit crazy when no-one had any answers. I saw his empty bed and concluded that he was dead."

"I guess I can understand that. How is he dealing with his illness?"

"Bravely. Better than I am. His attitude is that what can't be cured, must be endured. I don't want him to see that I've been crying. He doesn't need a wimpy mother before his surgery. I just got so scared. For him, and for myself. I don't want him to be in pain, and helpless. I want him to get stronger again. I can't let him go. Not now. Not ever."

"Does he talk about the full-blown AIDS?"

"No. He never complains. He just withdraws; he's more like his father than I realized. He hates being in here, though. The ward noises irritate him, and prevent him from sleeping. He feels threatened when the Alzeheimer patients from the adjoining ward wander in here, and he's alone. They have taken some of his clothing and his toiletries. He's a very private person, and he detests being imposed upon when he can't defend himself. He doesn't say much, but I can see the anger in his eyes, and hear the anguish in his voice."

"That is a concern. We try to maintain some type of vigil over them, but they're obstreperous and difficult to discipline. Their vocal noises are not pleasant, either. Does Michael show any actual progress?"

"A little. His fever has decreased because of the antibiotics. He seems interested in his music and videos now, and follows the conversations of his visitors. His responses are more like the Michael that we love--cryptic and cynical. He has a very keen, dry humour. You'd enjoy him, if you got to know him."

The intern nodded, and waited for me to talk again.

"He's communicating a lot better, really. You'll recall that he couldn't seem to generate a response to many of your questions. He was too sick. Those doctors who have the courtesy to address him directly, instead of asking me, get logical answers."

The doctor turned his head to one side, and said, "Is that a common practice, ignoring the AIDS patient?"

"Yes. It upsets Michael, and makes me furious. As soon as it starts I get agitated. It appears to me that his life has been discounted. Because he is terminally ill, they consider him already dead. Michael just smiles wearily and says, 'Don't worry about it Mom. There is no need.' NO NEED. He says that too much lately. He is not usually a submissive individual. It sounds as though he is quitting--giving up."

"You want him to keep fighting."

"You're damn right. Surely to God they can find a cure for this disease. They keep promising more research funding. Every other day they offer a new procedure for hope. Perhaps they are making promises which they cannot keep. It's one hell of a way to die, penalized because a person searched for a little love, a little comfort. No one should have to pay such a price."

"Is Michael homosexual?"

"Yes. But he's not certain that he got AIDS through sex. He told me that he's practiced safe sex, and not risked his life. He has too much to live for. He loves to travel, to study, to hope for a better world."

"How else do you think he could have contracted the disease?"

"In 1981 Michael had a double hernia operation. It's a congenital problem, acquired from his father, grandfather and grandmother. At twenty months of age, he had his initial double hernia operation in Hamilton. When they did the second operation here in Toronto, they found that his insides were a mess. They repaired the left side one day, and the right side the following day. He required three bags of blood. No blood was tested in Ontario in 1981. You probably know that it was not until 1985 that they screened for the virus.

Michael never really regained his strength after that operation. He went to Edmonton for his Co-operative Work sessions with the university six months later. He was hospitalized with hepatitis for three weeks, and we nearly lost him. I talked with the head nurse over the phone a few times, and I prayed like a maniac. For two days there was little hope. The horror of that comes back pretty quickly. I feel intuitively that it was the blood that he was given."

"Did he ever have any other STD's?"

"Sure he did. Homosexuals frequently have to contend with those things. He suffered with genital warts, herpes, and a few bouts of syphilis. I don't know whether or not he ever had gonorrhea. It just wasn't any of my business, so I never asked. Why do you ask? Do you think that the AIDS piggy-backs on STD's?"

NOT A TOTAL WASTE

"Not necessarily. But gay males who have STD's, who are promiscuous, have a lot higher rate of AIDS. Did Michael have one special relationship?"

"Oh, hell! I don't know. It's not my business. Still, I wished that he had someone special right now. Someone to cherish him-- to care about how ill he is. I know that he had a few relationships, but I didn't meet them. He certainly has the most remarkable friendships, at this time of his life. I've met the people that really matter to him, and they're fantastic. I'm grateful that they have been so kind to Michael and to me."

"What about drugs? Needles?"

"Who knows, really. I asked him once if he used needles, and he looked shocked. He said, "Never, Mother!" I believe him. He's probably had many social opportunities to use hash and coke. At one time he drank more than was healthy, but did not become addicted. He's a light social drinker, now. When we go out for dinner, he enjoys a fine dry martini, or a Caesar. I've never seen him intoxicated, nor have I seen him drink beer or ale. That doesn't mean that he doesn't imbibe those beverages. It's just that he basically seems to have avoided over-indulgences. He's not an angel, but he's not a reprobate, either. What difference does it make, exactly how he got AIDS? Would it change anything? HE HAS IT...and there's no cure."

"I'm sorry if my questions upset you. I guess that the more I see it happen, the more I try to analyze. If we could just know how to prevent it, or decrease it, in the future it could save lives."

"The way that less fat in the diet might decrease breast cancer? If more funds were available for research, perhaps we'd have had a cure by now. Mike tells me that there is an alarming projection that AIDS will become a heterosexual disease--a killer of children. Not enough is being done to stop AIDS. Nature may have started it, but our own ineptness is permitting it to steal lives. Political priorities need changing. How and when Mike got AIDS is of little consequence. If he'd known that the disease was out there, he would have taken the most care possible".

"Michael practiced safe sex?"

"We've talked about condoms, sterile needles and the practices of safe sex. I believe that he has used precautions. You have to remember that this disease was not understood, nor even publicized, when it first began to spread. No one considered those recent calculations that if you have one lover per year for six years, and so do all of your lovers, you could virtually have had sexual contact with 45,000 individuals. As a result, every sexually active person in the world, with more than one partner, is at risk. Marriage is no real guarantor of protection. Infected spouses provide no shield. Also, spontaneity can happen to anyone. Think of how many spur-of-the-minute sexual experiences which have resulted in unwelcome surprises. Michael has too much to live for, to die such a miserable death. He didn't select this disease. It chose him. It's a type of retrovirus, and it can hide for over a decade in the blood. Isn't that correct?"

"Yes, it is."

"I guess, unless someone that you love is affected by AIDS, you don't feel any panic about AIDS depopulating the world. You hear the nasty jokes about it, you read the headlines and scan some of the write-ups, but you don't dig for data. With this disease, everyone is going to be affected in one way or another. It's racing through the heterosexual community now like wildfire. They say that prostitutes are becoming younger and younger, as their customers search for an AIDS-free virgin. Teen-agers believe that they're immortal, and refuse to take precautions. You're either going to know somebody with it, or have someone close to you die."

"You've thought about this quite a lot."

"Yes, I have. I've learned that no-one is safe. This killer is stalking our families. The only prerequisite for the disease is that you must be human. We can't keep ignoring the facts. When Stephan, Michael's friend, died of AIDS-related pneumonia, I worried over when it would hit Michael full-force. There are a lot of other things to wonder about, too."

"Do you mean social relationship changes which he would have to contend with? Financial worries? What?"

"Sure. Some 'so-called friends' disappear. Once you are too ill to work full-time, or eventually not at all, money worries are very real. There are at least half a dozen of those opportunistic infections that can destroy you. They run the immune system down, and leave you physically and emotionally drained. Financial assistance isn't available, even if you can't work, until you are medically defined as an AIDS case."

"Welfare can be made available, can't it?"

"Stephan had to wait until he got a specific disease so that he could state that he had CDC-defined AIDS. Then he could get his doctor to provide a letter, so that he could apply for welfare. It takes time. He hated welfare."

"Do you mean he hated to take financial assistance?"

NOT A TOTAL WASTE 47

"He hated the red tape, and the shabby, demeaning way in which he was treated. He had to have his doctor fill out endless forms, for his employer and the social service system. He felt that he was burdening the doctor, and begging from society. He hated to grovel, as much as Michael does. When Stephan was so sick, Mike just said, "It's a no-win situation, Ma.""

"Perhaps it won't be that bad for Michael. He'll have learned how to get the help that he needs from the system."

"Michael has already had some rough experiences because of the homophobic attitudes of some of the social workers. There are some that seem to be right out of it, too often."

"Do you think it's because this is a relatively new disease, and they are inexperienced in dealing with it?"

"Maybe. Michael is not the only one who gets depressed, dealing with the public's paranoia. When you ask for help, and get shifted from one department to another without a good explanation, you feel as if you're being shafted. He's been too sick to make many demands. He said that he can smell the intolerance a mile away, when he deals with some of the social services. Maybe the disease makes him extra sensitive. Think about it. He's carrying a terminal disease. People generally hate anyone who admits to being gay. Familial disapproval frequently creates acute loneliness. Imagine it. They are dying, yet their families abandon them due to their own fear and pain. Society isolates the sick--and wishes that the contaminated person with AIDS would evaporate. No wonder Michael has been worried about his potential for any future at all."

"His doctors have provided the necessary support, though?"

"Yes, and we're grateful. You know, there's one aspect which I haven't thought about, insofar as medical treatment is concerned. Some of Mike's doctors are gay, but others are obviously straight. Wouldn't the public censure them, too, because they are predominantly treating patients with AIDS-related illnesses? I mean...it must take courage for any doctor to indicate a defiance of societal acceptance."

"There is that element. But in this profession, sincere dedication demands that those prejudicial considerations are just not a priority."

"But they also risk their lives. You'll soon have your own patients. You could catch AIDS from one of them."

"There is an infinitesimal risk, for any care giver."

"I guess on the other hand, a doctor could infect me, too."

"Also a minute chance, since so many precautions are undertaken. The world is not without hazards, wherever AIDS is involved. We recognize that."

"Whew. Not sure...that it makes me feel very secure. I have a friend who has purchased a dental drill head for her family's use each time that they have fillings. She is terrified that she can catch AIDS through unsanitary equipment in her dentist's office."

"This disease is complex, but I can tell you that experts are constantly trying to solve the riddle."

"The statistical evidence won't go away. The numbers of those who are becoming infected and dying from this killer disease are still climbing."

"Yes. That's true. I wish it weren't. I have lost a few friends from AIDS, too. No-one can turn a 'blind eye', since it is also locating prey among heterosexuals."

"It wrenches my heart--and my gut--that they die such a horrible death. They are discarded as they die because people are paranoid of the disease and its connotations. Michael told me of three of his friends who murdered themselves and died in seclusion. Their bodies were discovered by friends, remains cremated, and ashes blown to the winds. They have no gravestone, no marker, nothing left to indicate their existence. Their talents, skills and entities have been eliminated. They have been treated as a breed apart. It is unjust."

"I agree. Look, once you take Michael home, if you should need a doctor for some reason, you could page me. If there's something that is worrying you, or if Michael has some concerns, maybe I could help. My hours vary, but you could ask them to check the schedule. It doesn't matter what time you call during the night, when I am on duty. If I can help you or Michael, call me."

"Thanks. I know that you're very busy. Still, your offer means a lot to me."

CHAPTER SIX

The orderly maneuvered the wheelchair through the doorway and towards the bed. Michael smiled, "Hi, Mom," and nodded towards the young intern. He may have recalled his help in the Admissions Department. His countenance showed good will. The doctor left with the orderly. Michael got settled into his bed just as the assistant neurosurgeon arrived.

It took an hour to prepare Michael for the biopsy. The barbaric preparations took place in his own room, with me observing and sharing in his agony. My heart told me that I must stand beside Mike for however long it took to complete the surgery. I only prayed that I could borrow a portion of his courage. Starting at eleven o'clock, the doctor and the same Nursing Assistant who had bad-mouthed AIDS patients in the hall the day before, worked as a team.

Michael was positioned in the wheelchair again, and a contraption was placed onto his skull which would assist with the surgery. A local anaesthetic was injected into his skull in the front, back, and both sides. Four holes were bored into his head so that the measured steel rulers, set into the four-cornered wooden frame, could be contrived to give an accurate reading of the exact location of the brain lesions. It was critical that they entered the brain at the precise lesion area as indicated by the CAT scans and X-rays. Once this structure was in place, Michael was left sitting rigidly upright in the wheelchair.

The bedsores which had developed at the base of his tail bone were open and bleeding. He had so little flesh left to provide any cushion for the coccyx area while seated, that I wondered how he could remain stoic. The doctor left him in this rigid position to await the arrival of the orderly, who would take him to the operating theatre.

Michael was unable to lie back, and could not touch the cage which was anchored firmly into his skull. Blood dripped down his forehead, the sides and back of his head, whenever the wooden frame was slightly moved. No lunch was brought, and Michael grew steadily more exhausted.

Remaining seated in this position, without relief, was more than strenuous. It seemed to be a medieval type of punishment. He closed his eyes, and valiantly waited. I used a cloth to wipe the blood away from his eyes, but he neither winced nor moved. I grew more anguished as the afternoon progressed, but Michael showed incredible fortitude. By four o'clock he asked about the time, and admitted that he was very tired.

Privately, I wished that I could have had all of the surgeons involved sitting on the head of a pin, or roasting in hell, with Dr. Baker holding them all together. However, I clamped my mouth tightly and pretended to read an espionage novel.

At four-fifteen the orderly fetched Michael. He had sat still for five hours, and it would be four more hours before he would be returned to his bed. The lack of consideration shown to him left me outraged. I tried to eat, despite my fury, to retain my strength. My supper consisted of coffee, a biscuit and pudding. Penny, Lucy, Therese, Corey and Ted all appeared shortly after eight o'clock, expecting to find Michael convalescing in his room. They shared my vigil by chattering over the weather, current events, music and food. At eight-thirty Michael was wheeled down the hall unconscious, conveyed upon a gurney, with his head encased in a large white turban. I could not bear to watch the transference and stumbled away. Corey's hand was suddenly under my elbow. I reeled to face him.

NOT A TOTAL WASTE — 51

"Corey, I just can't. Oh God, I just can't. Is he all right? Tell me."
"He opened his eyes and spoke to Lucy. Take your time. I'll go back with you when you're ready."
"I'm sorry, Corey. I've behaved all day, but I don't have Michael's courage."
"It's all right. You're his mother."
"Okay, I'll try. Let's go and see how he feels."

He lay very quietly, but his eyes were open. He listened to his friends' conversations, and smiled slightly when I came beside his bed. We remained with him for about twenty minutes, until the night nurse arrived. She introduced herself and suggested that Michael required extra rest after his surgery. We realized that we should leave him, but accepted her suggestion with regret. I kissed him gently on the cheek, and we headed in a dishevelled gaggle towards the elevator. Corey dropped me off that evening. I phoned Bruce and Anna right away to let them know how Michael was doing, and then fell into a fitful slumber.

That night was filled with horrible apparitions and dreams. Mercifully, the morning sunlight woke me early. Anna drove over from Hamilton to take me to the hospital the following morning, and I was grateful for her company. The experiences of the previous day had left me emotionally and physically drained. We found Michael awake, but feverish again. He was glad to see his sister. They had always been close companions, and it was good to see his joy at her presence. She chatted for about half an hour, and then explained that she had some blueprints and supplies to pick up. Traffic on the Queen Elizabeth and 401 highways were heavier than usual due to a few accident tie-ups, so she left with a promise to return the following day.

Michael slept again after Anna left. Plans had been made for me to return home that week-end to return Sean and Jenni to their parents, but this trip hinged upon Michael's reaction to the surgery and the new medication. I went for a short walk around the grounds, picked up some extra tooth-paste, mouth wash and shaving cream for Michael, and returned to his room.

Dr. Baker was standing beside Michael's bed, and Mike seemed agitated. I held my breath and tried hard not to intervene.

My concern was that something negative had been discovered during the surgery.

"What do you mean, you won't have the surgery again?"
"Exactly what I told you before. There is no need."
"Oh, come on. You've had worse pain than this in your life, haven't you?"
"Sure, but not by my own choice."
"The tissue sample was normal. We can only conclude that the surgeons have missed the right spot. We'll have to go in to obtain tissue from the surrounding area for our testing purposes."
"No bloody way."
"You're being unreasonable. Perhaps your mother can talk some sense into you."

I saw the pain in Michael's eyes, and watched him turn his face to the wall as his eyes brimmed over. I felt a similar welling up of anger. I wanted him better, but I also felt an innate need to protect him from Dr. Baker's decision to plan a second bout of surgery. I spoke as slowly and calmly as I could muster.

"Dr. Baker, Michael feels that this is an unnecessary imposition. The error made in obtaining the tissue sample has nothing to do with his desire to refuse any further surgery. Have you not checked his chart, as he previously requested?"

She stared at me, amazed that I would not support her intent to do a second brain biopsy. I stood serenely, indicating a bravado which I did not possess. Her eyes blazed as she spoke,

"You want his health to improve, don't you? How can this occur without additional testing?"
"I don't know. I wish I did. I'm sorry, but I respect Michael's decision. He has refused any life-extending procedures."

She swished out of the room. Michael looked over at me and gave just a hint of a weary smile, and then closed his eyes. I walked slowly up to his bed, and patted him lovingly on his hand.

"Michael, this is the date that you should have your Pentamadine breathing treatment. I checked with the nurse, and she ordered the

NOT A TOTAL WASTE

mobile kit from the clinic downstairs. I saw it on the counter when I came in. Shall I get it for you and help you to use it now?"

He cleared his throat, and replied, "Okay, Mom. I'll try."

The availability of this medication at Metro clinics had been a recent contribution by a concerned physician to the AIDS community. Results indicated its value for the prevention of AIDS-related pneumonia. The inhalation of the Pentamadine spray coated the lungs and reduced the impact of secondary infection. Michael had been going regularly to the Rosedale Clinic for his appointments. He had a racking, chronic cough that did not seem to be alleviated by any medication, but had not had pneumonia. When I went to the nursing station to pick up the kit, Dr. Baker held Michael's chart in her hand.

"Come over here, please," she requested softly. I stood beside her and waited. "I see he has a Living Will here, and your Power of Attorney. I'm certain that you realize that the Living Will is not recognized as a legal document in Ontario. No doctor has to comply with these wishes. That's all that they are. Patient's wishes. And I assume that you are the doctor that is referred to here?"

"Yes."

"Well, what does that mean, exactly? That you're a medical doctor, and therefore have the authority to over-rule every decision that is made towards fostering Michael's recovery?"

"Oh God, no. I'm only a Ph.D. doctor. It's all a crock of shit. My education doesn't help. None of it can save my only son."

My voice choked and my eyes filled. I wanted to run, but I was afraid of heading smack into a wall. The complete uselessness of everything that I had ever accomplished in my life, hit home hard.

She reached her hand out and steadied me. "Oh, I see. I understand. Because I can't really help my own kids, either. And this disease takes away so many incredible young people. Always at the prime of their lives. There's only so much that anyone can do."

I stared at her. Her eyes, also, were overflowing. She lowered her head, wiped her eyes, and forged slowly down the hall. Rooted to the spot, I watched her leave. I fully realized that this tough little doctor was a wife, mother, and a medical doctor with a gruelling work load. Her demeanor told different stories, now. She only appeared tough as a protective measure, for herself and her patients. She had a prickly-pear exterior, but internally she was genuinely loving and caring. With the stress which she had to experience each day, it was amazing that she had not already suffered burn-out. Now, shame tugged at my conscience. My prior frustration over her perfectionism was not a comfortable memory. I seemed to have a different perspective, now. I felt secure in the knowledge that Dr. Baker would do her very best to prolong Michael's health and life.

I wondered whether she felt fear over the professional risks engendered from treating AIDS patients. She had family obligations too, and her work with HIV seropositive patients must worry her about potential consequences of exposure to the disease. Would Dr. Baker, who worked almost exclusively with AIDS clients, suffer negative responses from society or her colleagues due to prejudice against her practice? She must cope daily with stresses of HIV care and the turbulent progression of the disease. She had shown me clear frustration and pessimism over her increasing volume of AIDS patients.

Because section VI of the American Medical Association's Code of Ethics supports the fact that any doctor "is free, except in emergencies, to choose whom to serve", Dr. Baker obviously offered her knowledge in a most professional affirmation of caring for the sick. She did not flee from the performance of her duties, any more than a fireman, soldier or policeman. Did she believe that AIDS was God's punishment to homosexuals for their immorality? Her conduct was professional, despite the overwhelming stress related to this care.

The leisurely pace at which society has handled the AIDS crisis will likely result in an epidemic of pandemic proportions. Both Medical doctors and their AIDS patients need protection from the developing medical, ethical and legal concerns. Maybe as the number of AIDS patients increases, homophobia will decrease. Negative attitudes and ethical issues related to AIDS patients and their medical teams could be alleviated through expansive educational training. Anti-discrimination laws require revision to include the AIDS patient, in addition to the handicapped. Disabiity insurance must include the occupational risks of treating AIDS

NOT A TOTAL WASTE 55

patients. With gratitude, I realized that Michael's doctors illustrated the type of dedication and moral integrity essential to caring for HIV affected individuals.

After clearing away the Pentamadine equipment for Michael, changing his sheets and nightgown, I left him to rest. Sitting in the coffee shop, I mused over the morning's happenings. I had vented raw anger towards Dr. Baker, and now I had to learn to forgive myself, too. My reaction had been normal, considering the stress which I was experiencing. Learning to let go of the guilt and to be kind to myself, would take considerable effort for a demanding type A personality. I was probably harder on myself, and more critical, than anyone else. Life's lessons never came easily.

Throughout that week, Michael's temperature varied from near normal to panic alert. His condition fluctuated constantly, and I was afraid that he would literally starve to death. He was so frail. However, he had a few good days towards the end of the following week, so I risked flying home to bring back the grandchildren. When I climbed the stairs, the children rushed to give me hugs and kisses. Bruce stood at the top of the stairs waiting to envelop me in a bear hug. I heard both dogs bark behind the louvred kitchen doors. Happily, I opened the door and called Molly and Mandii to come and get their kisses. Molly, a one-year old golden labrador had been selected by Michael from a local breeder, on his last visit home. She wriggled every-which-way and produced a crazy grin that made Sean and Jenni giggle. Mandii lay behind the kitchen table, and when she tried to stand, she fell forward with a scream and a crash to the floor. She lay there looking at me moaning, and I stared.

"My God, what's happened to her?"
"She's been to the vet, Maria. We can't do anything about it. There's some damage to the right shoulder. It seems to be related to the car accident that she had as a puppy, long before we bought her. The bone is disintegrating. The needles and painkillers can't touch it."

I ran to her and sat on the floor beside her. Mandii was a huge German Shepherd that I thought of as "my" dog. I had bought her from a graduate student who couldn't keep her any longer. She was the one who comforted me, listened to my woes and licked away my tears without walking away. Now, she lay unable to stand.

"You'll have to put her down, Bruce. She can't live like this. Why did you wait? She's in so much pain."
"I just couldn't do that right now, without you seeing her first. Not with Michael's illness, too. Is that really what you want?"
"Yes. As soon as possible. No dog should have to tolerate that kind of suffering."
"You're right. I'll take her to the doctor tomorrow."

Euthanasia seemed to be the right thing to do for a dog in extreme agony, yet our civilization would not agree on the same consideration or opportunity for a human being. The incongruity made me dizzy. I would be criticized if I let Mandii struggle for her existence, and society would easily condone her relief through death. But if an individual realized that the quality of his own life was so inadequate that he could not face any further pain and begged to end it through his own means, a furor resulted. Surely the ones to complain the loudest against permitting a loved one to determine their own fate, were the ones who had either never experienced excruciating, unending pain, or they loved selfishly.

Michael was constantly on my mind, even as I looked at Mandii. He had refused the Hickman catheter. That device would have permitted the insertion of medicine and food intravenously through a small tube attached to a vein in his chest. As I watched Mandii, panting and glassy-eyed from pain, I remembered how Michael had stated that he did not want tubes stuck out every orifice of his body. He made me promise that no ventilator would insistently inflate his lungs, when they were too weary to function. Life-sustaining measures were not part of Michael's plans, and I felt morally and ethically bound to respect those wishes. If his life came to the point where it could no longer succeed, I must have the strength and sufficient love to let him go gently into the night. I would have to borrow some of his spirit. Michael was brave beyond measure, and I vowed that his decision would be respected--there would be no further invasive treatment.

Anna met our plane, and we all went straight to the hospital to check on Michael's condition. He seemed flushed and disoriented, but he did recognize the children. He adored them both and was thrilled at their visit. Because of an infection in the larynx, his speech was halting and scratchy. Anna and the children stayed only ten minutes, and then said, "Take care of yourself, Uncle Mike. We love you", and kissed his cheek. Anna kissed his cheek, too, and blinked back tears. They were quickly gone, and the room was quiet once more.

David entered, his arms loaded with flowers, magazines and music tapes.

"Hi, how was the flight?"

"Not bad at all. Last time, someone had played handball, tossing my plane from cloud to cloud. This trip was excellent. You just missed Anna and the children. They were here to see Michael."

"You'd appreciate that, Mike. Has your fever been reduced at all?"

Michael did not answer, but looked steadily at the ceiling before he wearily closed his eyes. Busily, I arranged David's flowers in the clear-crystal vase which he had bought. The tapes and magazines were placed on Michael's bedside table. David stood beside Michael, willing him to wake up, to speak, to react. I shook my head and pointed towards the doorway. We closed the door softly behind us, and David placed his hand on my elbow to guide me towards the elevator.

"Where can we talk?"

"Let's go to the lobby. It's got some comfortable chairs, and it's large enough so that we can isolate ourselves and gain privacy. On the way I want to show you a funny stuffed puppy that I saw in the gift shop. If it's still there later, I want to get it for Michael. It has that Michael look--you know, that sort of half smile and the strange staring eyes that seem to plead, "Why ME? Can't someone fix this?"

David laughed, "You mean the way he looked when you burned the chicken that time? And when the pumpkin pie wasn't cooked in the centre? Good idea!"

"You would remember my cooking problems...good thing that you surprised us that afternoon with the quarter-pounders with cheese."

We relaxed and felt as though some pressure had been removed, somehow.

"So, tell me about Michael," David urged.

We talked for over an hour. Michael was trying to handle supper when we returned. He had progressively lost sensation in his right side throughout the past three months, and it had become worse since his surgery. His right hand would not function properly, and now it was completely devoid of any feeling. He had difficulty manipulating his right foot in walking. I had teased him about staggering like a "drunken sailor", and told him that he had been the first, after four generations of nautical men, to become dysfunctional without the help of the legal "tot of rum". He had given me a cursory grunt and not spoken of it again. Now, I watched him ineffectively spilling soup against the side of his mouth and down the front of his nightgown. He had tried to eat the sandwich, but the bread was too stale for him to swallow. It lay discarded on his tray. Gently, I took the spoon, and fed him his pudding and tea. David chatted for a short time, and left with a promise to drop in the following evening.

Michael wanted to watch television for the first time in quite awhile, so we shared his delight at watching Picard's STAR TREK. This was a favourite treat for him!

"Mom, did you ever notice the change in the Intro?"
"No. What do you mean?"
"They're now asexual. They don't say, 'To boldly go where no man has gone before.' It's been changed."
"Hmmph. You mean sexual discrimination has been averted?"
"Yes. You'll be pleased to notice that now they say, 'to boldly go where no one has gone before.' What do you think of that?"
"Guess there's hope for the space world, after all."

We both laughed. Seeing him able to smile made me forget my own exhaustion, and I could feel myself relax.

A young intern entered the room, and asked Michael how he was responding to treatment. We had never seen this doctor before, but Michael told him that his projectile vomiting and explosive diarrhea were not abating. His fever still ranged from 101 to 104, or more. The intern nodded, and said he'd check Michael's chart. When he came into the room again, he ignored me and went directly to Michael.

NOT A TOTAL WASTE

"The medication seems normal for your illness. Have you been travelling much?"
"All over the globe."
"Anywhere in particular recently?"
"How recently?"
"Within the last three or four months."
"Yes, I was in France for a few weeks, about three months ago. Had planned to get to Amsterdam, but took sick in Paris."
"Oh, Paris. It's been a hotbed for toxoplasmosis."
"What's that?"
"Well, it's a disease of man, dogs, cats--and certain other mammals. It's caused by a parasitic microorganism. It especially affects the nervous system."
"Does it cause diarrhea, and these related fevers? Sore throat? Vomiting? Would it complicate my coordination problems?"
"Yes, it could."
"What can I do about it? How can you test for it?"

The intern looked thoughtful, and said, "I'd like to look into this a bit more. There is a powerful antibiotic that can be used. Its side effects can be deleterious, so it must be evaluated consistently, and used with caution. Have you had CAT scans? Were there any lesions in the brain?"

I couldn't sit still any longer. I was literally shaking with excitement.

"Do you mean that if he had a brain biopsy, and no cancerous lesions were found, that it is possible that the lesions seen on CAT scans and X-rays could be due to this infection? How noxious is this drug?"
"I think it is possible. It would need more testing."
"How can you fight an infection like that and win? You know that AIDS patients can catch infections that don't give a healthy person's immune system any problem. The public gets so paranoid about catching AIDS, but they have no idea how much more dangerous it is for a person living with AIDS to catch viral or bacterial infections from them. Their immune system can't fight back."
"Yes, that's true."
"If he has toxoplasmosis, how fast can we get him better?"
"Hey, hold it. Let's find out first if he does have it."

"How can you do that?"
"Well, how long have you been ill, Michael?"
"Oh, let's see. After I got back from Paris, I took it easy. Then, three weeks ago, a neighbour's cat was hit by a car. I took her to the vet, and she had to be destroyed. She scratched my arm, and it got infected, but it didn't seem too serious. I guess I haven't been so well, since then. The fevers and nausea started first."
"Toxoplasmosis can definitely create lesions throughout the body in an AIDS patient, Michael. I'm going to check with the resident medical team, and get back to you later this evening."
"Well, Mom? Shall we expect miracles?" Michael grinned at me.

My throat felt choked with emotion, so that I could not reply. I smiled happily, and nodded my head in agreement. Miracles...we would both expect miracles. Michael and I were animated about the possibilities which the intern had explained, and the hope for a solution to the secondary infection. I was certain that this pernicious infection was devastating his body. I knew that cancer was still a definite possibility, and that these could be cancerous lesions. Yet, my gut-level instinct told me that there could also be hope for a treatable disease. If a cure was not available, at least we could aspire to extend his life.

That evening I was bathing Michael's body with rubbing alcohol again, desperately trying to bring down his fever. He was in and out of consciousness when the intern returned with three other doctors. Michael could not respond to their questions. Shakily, I tried to give the best answers that I could, but my mind was concentrating on Michael's weakened body. That night, an antibiotic was administered, and within four days it was deleted from his drug tray. His appetite developed and he seemed alert. This was more like the Michael that we loved. His cynical, dry humour surprised the doctors and nurses, and delighted his loved ones. He was back!

By the end of that week we realized that Dr. Baker was on vacation, but that Michael would be released with home care, and visiting Victorian Order of Nurses. The home care would be provided for a limited duration, which could be extended, if necessary. Their tasks would be to do laundry, meals, and bed changes. The VON would monitor medications, his rate of

NOT A TOTAL WASTE 61

progress, and general level of health. They would check on him each morning, and gradually reduce their number of calls until he was functioning independently again. Delighted, we prepared for his departure from the hospital. Michael shaved himself while I packed his few belongings. His plush puppy and teddy-bear were tucked safely beside his gifts and toiletries. He stood beaming at me, ready to go home. His blue jeans hung loosely on his frame, and his T-shirt seemed to belong to someone else. It didn't matter; we would soon fatten him up at home.

Once I had Michael seated in the wheelchair, the nurse came with release papers and other documents which had to be signed. Paula, the hospital social worker, came to say good-bye, and asked to talk with me alone. I didn't like to leave Michael sitting unwatched in the chair, so I guided him towards the bed. He did not mind resting on top of the bed for a short time. While the nurse checked his temperature, I went to the next room with Paula.

"Here is a card, Maria, with my telephone number. Don't hesitate to contact me at any time of the day or night. I have a beeper, and the call can be forwarded."

"I doubt if I would need it, but I appreciate your thought."

"Would you like someone from the Casey House Hospice, to call on you? Or a member of the clergy?"

I looked at her, and wondered why she was taking my time with this now. "No, I don't feel any need for that. However, if you have the telephone number for the Persons With AIDS Foundation, or the AIDS Committee of Toronto, I'd appreciate having either of them. Michael might like to have someone visit him, or need to obtain information. Once Michael is well again, I will have to return home by the second week in August to prepare for school. It would comfort me to know that he is not lonely. This ostracism of society is tough to handle; Michael spends too much time isolated."

Paula complied with that request, but insisted that I take her card, as well. She said, "Dealing with death is very difficult, especially since you are alone with Michael in the city. You may need someone to talk to, or I could refer you to a counsellor. Perhaps Michael will require a palliative care counsellor as well, in order to come to terms with his situation."

I stared at her with mounting incredulity. Who in the hell can ever fully come to terms with their own terminal illness? And what kind soul is suddenly going to wave a magic wand and make us feel better about it? Did she think we were not fully conscious of where this disease would lead us, in the end? And when I can no longer reach out and touch him, see his smile, hear his contagious laughter, what words will help me then? Who will bring Michael back to me? Are there truly bandaids for shredded hearts? I felt anger at her blandish sweetness. Had she ever really suffered like this, watching a beloved die?

This disease was like no other. It didn't cause a daily decline, bit by bit, like cancer. This was often called Lazarus' disease, because the patient could seem so close to death, and yet somehow survive. AIDS caused an emotional roller coaster for patient and loved ones--wondering if the remission would last for just a little longer. Didn't she think that I had been pre-grieving for months now, watching Michael lose his strength, freedom and dignity? I gave a quivering kind of laugh, which denied any potential of Michael's demise, and backed out of the room. When I got back to Michael, I patted his arm, and gently asked,

"How're you doing, Son?"
"I just want to get out of this place, and back to my own apartment, and my own bed, Ma. I want to get home."
"Well, then, since all the papers are finished with--let's blow this place."

I wheeled him around to push the chair through the door, and found it blocked by Dr. Baker's colleague. She was taking care of all patients, in Dr. Baker's absence.

"Did they come up to see you from downstairs?"
"No, who?"
"I mean from the laboratory. Didn't they tell you the news?"
Michael and I stared at her, willing her to get to the final point of her questions. I could taste the bile rising in my throat from tension.

"The recent CAT scans, since you began taking the antibiotic, have indicated that the lesions have begun to dissipate. You were

NOT A TOTAL WASTE 63

right, Michael. You are battling toxoplasmosis, not cancer. Isn't that exciting?"

To say that it was exciting is putting it mildly. Michael and I were literally sailing down that hall in a matter of minutes, carrying the nurses good wishes behind us. The doctor had provided us with prescriptions for potent antibiotics, and a warning to watch for highly contagious mouth thrush. When the "big gun" antibiotics are used, sometimes the fungus infections develop rampantly. Michael was already ingesting so many different drugs. Caution would be demanded. They must be divided into daily requirements, placed into little plastic cubicles and sorted with real care. Four times a day, Michael would have to be assured that he had received the correct balance of medications. These would leave him nauseated, confused, and with an impaired sense of balance. Hopefully, they would lead him towards an eventual recovery.

We rode home to his apartment by taxi, our eyes weeping and our mouths smiling. The three week stay in the hospital had been a gruelling interim, that was now behind us. With luck and lots of prayers, we were going to succeed. Michael reached over and patted my hand. We grinned at each other like a pair of silly, happy fools. We were determined to squeeze as much pleasure as possible from what remained of his precious life. Michael arrived at his apartment by one-thirty on that last Saturday in July, 1990, and slept for fifteen hours. He was home--in his own bed.

SECTION TWO

CHAPTER ONE

Dawn would not come quickly enough for me, the following morning. I was so excited about Michael being home, in his own bed again, that I peeked in on him frequently. Around four o'clock in the morning, the noise of my opening his bedroom door must have inadvertently awakened him. He stirred, and slowly turned to face me.

"Morning, honey. I'm sorry to wake you. It's only four-ish. Are you too warm?"

"No, not really," he replied with a scratchy-sounding voice.

"Michael, I found a small fan in the kitchen, which could fit on your window sill. Do you want me to plug it in?"

"No, Mom. I'm okay. In fact, could I have my own duvet back? The fingers on my right hand keep getting caught in this thermal blanket."

I stepped forward, and realized that I should have placed a sheet on top of the blue thermal blanket, in order to prevent his fingers from catching in the holes. Before he returned home I had removed and packed away David's elegant duvet set, and replaced the bedding. Therese and Lucy had spent an afternoon shopping for my listed items of bedclothes. Fitted plastic and quilted cotton underpads had a thick, dog-toothed foam pad placed over them, and flannel sheeting covered all of that. I had hoped to relieve Michael's bedsores in this manner, and effectively protect the new mattress. Due to the summer heat, I had removed his favourite jade-green duvet, but now he seemed to be trembling from cold.

"Michael, let me help you to have a warm shower, and I'll freshen up your bed. Can you manage that, dear?"
"I'm sure that I can, Ma."

He struggled to his feet, and I removed both diaper and surgical gown. I had discovered the gown inside the large box containing rubber gloves, face masks and diapers, provided for us by the hospital when we signed out. Michael did not own pyjamas, and I thought that the surgical gown would keep him from getting a chill during the night.

I saw instantly what a terrible error I had made. The impermeable fabric had been designed to protect against the contamination of bodily fluids. Because of this, it had not permitted Michael's perspiration to be absorbed. The urine spillage had collected in a rank pool against his skin. Due to urine scalding and night sweating, his torso was now a reddened mass of heat rash and blisters.

He stood frail and trembling before me, so I rapidly grabbed his terrycloth bathrobe to wrap around him. I led him to the shower, and gave him his privacy. The offensive gown and diapers were dumped unceremoniously into the triple layers of green garbage bags, sprayed with chlorine bleach and secured with a twist tie. My anger, at my own stupidity, choked me. I tried desperately to seem outwardly calm, as I changed his bedding. Once Michael was showered, diapered and dressed in the largest pure-cotton GAP T-shirt that he owned, I tucked him back into bed. I asked if he'd like to have a cup of hot milk.

"That would be great, Mom. I'm more comfortable now."
"Michael, I'm so sorry. You're urine burnt, have a heat rash, and freezing your ass off--all at once. This is the nurse from hell, here. I may as well have wrapped you in plastiwrap. Please forgive me."
"Nothing to get hung up about, Mom. I'm still here."

His blue eyes sparkled when I gave him the warm milk, and soon he slept again. However, I did not settle down for the rest of that night. Self-recriminations attacked me for hours. I belittled my efforts at home nursing, and wished that I'd had the forethought to have taken some prior training. It was obvious that these requisite skills, which I had taken for granted, were not part of human nature. The First Aid and Pulmonary Resuscitation courses which I had completed two months previously, had been a wise move. I had expected perfection from myself, and I had "messed up". I was no SUPERNURSE. What other blunders would I make? Was I more a hindrance than a help? Michael was certainly too ill to adapt to my mistakes in judgment. I simply could not forgive myself.

Just before ten o'clock, I gently woke Michael to ensure that he received his first medication and his breakfast. He gamely tackled juice, cereal, boiled egg, toast and tea. When he was tidied up and back into bed, I told him that I'd go to the corner laundromat and then shop for groceries on the way back. He expected to sleep for a few hours, so I got moving. I hated to leave him unattended for any length of time.

When I returned, he was still asleep. Rather than disturb him, I thought it a propitious time to hurry over to the Eaton's Centre. Michael needed some good cotton night-shirts. With the Victorian Order of Nurses representative, the homemaker and his friends expected to visit, he just couldn't parade around in diapers and T-shirts. Half a dozen men's nightshirts should carry him over from one laundry to the next. He must have an extra terrycloth housecoat, too. His Japanese black silk robe was too costly to dry clean, despite its comfortable sensation against his skin. One over-sized terrycloth wrap was not adequate. The heavy fabric took forever to dry, even at the laundromat.

As I stepped from the apartment, Anna surprised me. I was so thrilled to see her, that I hugged her too tightly. She had grown nearly as tall as I, but was finer-boned. Her hair was light blond, skin of dewy porcelain and clear blue eyes. She said that I was biased, whenever I told her that she was lovely. Her disposition was stable, and her personal feelings were forever imperturbable. She held her emotions in check constantly, and wore a bright cheery countenance for the world to see. I've always adored her, but felt a little in awe of her intangible self-reliance.

NOT A TOTAL WASTE

Her grooming courses had paid dividends; she had developed into an attractive, willowly woman.

"Mom, where are you headed?" she asked, once I had stopped hugging her.
"Oh, Anna, Michael had a rough time last night. It was my fault. I put one of those surgical gowns on him, in case he got a chill while he slept. The damn thing couldn't absorb his sweat or urine. He's got a body rash and his fever went sky high again."
"Should you leave him alone?"
"He's still sleeping. I was on my way over to Eaton's to locate some cotton nightshirts. He needs to look sophisticated, when people visit. He can't go to the can wearing a diaper and T-shirt."
Anna stared at me, grinned and shook her head in amusement. "Mike's this sick--and you worry about his dignity. Funny Mother! Come on, I'll drive you there. My car is just down the block. That way you can get back to him faster, and we can all have tea together. I have to submit a quote and pick up extra blueprints for Bernie. Let's hurry."

I tried to rush, but felt out of breath and a little wobbly. My heart tends to beat arrhythmically when under extreme stress or exhaustion, due to a congenital mitral valve problem. It has always been this way, and the best medicine is rest and relaxation--obviously not available for awhile. The sharp pain in the chest and light-headed feeling is not new, and was called a heart murmur by a doctor in Toronto years ago. It never frightens me, but it impedes my movements by slowing me down. I regulated my breathing carefully for a few moments, while I kept following Anna to the car. The pain was a warning for me to get sufficient sleep that night, or I wouldn't be capable of assisting Michael. Tension can do strange things, physically, emotionally and mentally, to those under duress. I was thoroughly exhausted, and would have to recognize these symptoms sooner. I could not risk my own health, since Michael was dependent upon my help.

We located six beautiful cotton nightshirts in the men's department at Eaton's. They were distinctive. Some had pin-stripes, tartans, or pastel hues. Anna and I returned to Michael quickly with these treasures, and hoped that he would approve of the tasteful styles and colours. He was in a deep, drugged sleep. I gently woke him, since it was time for his lunch and Anna wanted to visit with him. He agreed to wear one of the multi-green, striped shirts.

While he changed, I noticed that the bed sores on his coccyx bone were open wounds. The skin on his elbows, knees and ankles were cracked and bleeding, from being rubbed against the hospital sheets. His skin was very sensitive to the chlorine bleach used as a disinfectant. Because of his fevers, his body was dehydrated and his skin was peeling. Any pressure spots, since he had so little flesh covering his bones, were prone to scaling and splitting. Before he put on his fresh diaper and new executive-style nightshirt, I slipped on rubber gloves and slathered the Polysporin antibiotic cream onto his tailbone sores. A Clinique deep moisturizer was used on his arms, legs, neck and face. He winced, and pulled back a bit. I realized that he hated to be touched so familiarly, and I apologized for intruding. I concentrated on stepping back, to give him more personal space, as I applied the moisturizer. In tending Michael, I learned to put aside my own bashfulness, and just pushed forward to complete the necessary tasks. His reticence was indicative of his shyness. Because I respected that, I said little, moved quickly, and tried to efficiently complete those tasks which would permit him to rest better.

Anna stayed for soup, sandwiches and tea, and happily entertained Michael with anecdotes about Sean and Jenni. He enjoyed her visit, snorted with laughter a few times, and consumed most of his lunch. Watching them both sharing little stories and communicating with such affection was a pleasure for me. He didn't see Anna often enough. Her responsibilities kept her busy juggling time as wife, mother, chauffeur, business-partner, housekeeper-- the usual, irreplaceable woman. Nevertheless, he missed her and frequently asked about her, when the interval between visits was long.

After Anna left, Michael slept. He was still worn out from getting resettled in his own apartment. Having him back home, as an invalid, created some new problems for me regarding safety factors. Because of his illness, his needs had considerably altered. Besides the caution required in administering his medication, some unanticipated structural adaptations were essential. David purchased and installed stainless-steel safety guard rails, which reduced Michael's risk of falling in the bathtub. He cut back the kitchen cupboard doors above the narrow side-counter, and installed Kim's microwave oven snugly underneath. This helped me to prepare or warm food for Michael rapidly, retaining more

NOT A TOTAL WASTE

nutrients. Not being the world's best cook, I appreciated that addition to the kitchen.

The ancient, noisy refrigerator in the apartment had an inadequate closure seal around the door. It needed continual defrosting, manually, and I did not feel secure about the temperature control. We purchased a small apartment-sized freezer which maintained a dependable temperature. Concern for potential salmonella infections was legitimate. These could have caused Michael acute gastroenteritis, or food poisoning. He already had enough problems with nausea, vomiting and diarrhea. Because he was debilitated, food not kept cold enough in the older refrigerator was hazardous. His inability to swallow or digest many foods resulted in a restricted appetite range, and forewarned of malnutrition.

David brought heavy duty gloves, cooking utensils for the microwave oven, new sponge mops and cleaning supplies. We were grateful for the extra bedding, towels, and stocked shelves of groceries. It was fairly easy for me to pick up milk, eggs, bread and a few extras at the corner store, but I couldn't carry too much home. The actual cleaning of the apartment took more of my time, because I was concerned that Michael could catch some additional viral, bacterial or chemical infection. I used chlorine bleach on every surface, twice a day, to protect him. I was not paranoid about catching an infection from Michael. My real fear was that in his weakened condition, he was not strong enough to fight any new microbes which I could accidently introduce.

While Michael was incontinent, the bed was changed a minimum of three times a day. Additional flannel sheets, folded in half and laid underneath his buttocks, were changed more frequently. Soiled linens were placed in large orange garbage bags, and tied, until I could get to the laundromat. I also bagged Michael's diapers, but these were "triple-bagged", and sealed carefully. Because of the Metro regulations, they could not be put outside until the morning of collection. These tended to pile up in the kitchen on the steps which led to the patio. On the first Sunday night that Michael was home, the summer heat in the kitchen was horrendous. I scrubbed the steps and the floors, after placing the diaper garbage bags on the patio. Needless to say, I was tired by eleven that night, and overlooked bringing the bags back inside.

Around four o'clock the following morning, I heard a strange shuffling, snorting kind of sound. Most of the windows were open about a hand-span in height. Michael had installed large screws into the window frame which prevented the windows from being raised above that distance. I checked to see that Michael was all right, and then followed the noises of scratching and rustling. It seemed to emanate from the area of the kitchen window.

The noises persisted for a few moments, so I reached for the wooden spoon. I thought that any animals trying to get into the diaper bags might be alarmed by a sudden noise. I had no idea if animals could get AIDS from touching contaminated diapers, but I was distraught at the thought. After I banged the spoon sharply against the window ledge, I shouted, "SCAT". Suddenly, with a loud smack, a shape hurled itself at the large kitchen window, and clung onto the screen. The noise terrified me. I stepped backwards and made a strangled sound. All of this nocturnal racket awakened Michael. He said, "What is it, Mom?" I didn't reply, but quickly turned on the kitchen light. This illuminated the patio. To my complete amazement, besides the large raccoon which still clung to the screen, there were seven more. These were not your Algonquin Park cuties, but were the toughest, best-fed looking group of gangsters I'd ever seen. The huge ball of fur jumped down from the screen, but another flew at the bathroom window. I promptly shut both windows, turned off the light in the kitchen, and ran down the hall to Michael's room. In my terror, I forgot that he was convalescing, and I leaped onto the bed beside him. Michael reached his hand up to turn on the bedside lamp, squinted down at this shaking mass beside him, and said, "Mom, what's wrong?" I took a few deep gulps of air, and responded,

"Oh, Michael, there is an army of eight raccoons on the back porch. They've been trying to open the diaper bags, but because I have everything tightly sealed and triple-bagged, they can't open them. They can't even tear them. And they're mad at me because I tried to chase them away by banging the wooden spoon onto the window ledge."

Michael started to grin, and said, "They can't get in, Mother. They can't hurt you in here!"

NOT A TOTAL WASTE 73

I looked up at him, and he appeared serene and in control of the situation. He sat propped up against his pillows, steadily staring at this "nut case". I quivered like an aspen during a windstorm, and then convulsed with nervous laughter. The situation was totally ridiculous. A true Northwestern Ontario native wouldn't be terrified of a gang of marauding raccoons--under normal circumstances. Michael said, "Here, give me your hand. Poor little Mommy. Afraid of those big bad city beggers". We both snorted and giggled and, when my heart had stopped racing, I turned out his light and went back to my futon. Michael never referred to that escapade in the morning, and I was grateful. Needless to say, the garbage was collected without incident. I did not make the same mistake of leaving garbage on the back patio overnight.

CHAPTER TWO

The first morning that the VON nurse arrived, she came about an hour earlier than we had expected. Apparently the front door buzzers were malfunctioning again, so we had not realized that she was outside. About eight-thirty our sleep was interrupted by,

"Yoohoo. Yoohoo. Michael. Are you in there? Michael. It's the nurse. Please come and let me in. COME AND GET ME!"

I jumped to my feet and stood still for a few seconds, trying to figure out what had happened. For certain, that was no raccoon. I managed to get up the stairs to the front door of the apartment house, in my short summer nightgown, and quickly let her into Michael's ground-floor suite. She was really a charming person, who loved to laugh. Michael enjoyed the back and leg rubdowns, which toned his weakened muscles.

She seemed to make the whole world vibrate with good humour, and we were enthralled with her. Each day that she came, she would write copiously in a journal, relegated to a shelf of Michael's bookcase. I continued to unobstrusively study those reports, since they provided an accurate and expert opinion of how well Michael was functioning. My visits to Michael were generally every two or three week-ends, and those reports provided a detailed outline as to whether he was up, dressed or asleep when she arrived,

NOT A TOTAL WASTE

what he had been eating, which medications he was still ingesting, and a general overview of his health. The nurse continued to keep track of Michael for six weeks, and then this service was withdrawn. Michael's health had improved sufficiently that he no longer required regular nursing surveillance.

The home maker's assistance was also available for a limited interim. The initial woman that arrived on that Monday was a soft-spoken, seemingly shy person. Her duties had been outlined as meals, dishes, shopping, laundry, and tidying up the apartment. She would be expected to wash the bathroom daily, and sponge-mop the floors. In other words, she would take over the tasks which I was doing, presently. It meant that I would have time for other duties such as banking, medical appointments, extra shopping, or just enjoying Michael's company. Relaxation time for me would be a bonus.

The first day she prepared his meals, did the dishes, baked a lemon pie, chatted up a storm, and tidied up the kitchen cupboards. She had decided that the spices should be sorted according to age, with duplicates discarded. The balance of that day she moved the cupboard contents from one shelf to another. The New York steak which I had purchased for Michael was cooked to a tough, shoe-leather consistency, the fresh vegetables boiled so long that they had lost their colour, and the potatoes were not baked in the centre. She had used the gas oven during that sweltering day in August, but Michael made an effort to eat, anyway. I assumed that such inept results were due to first day nervousness, and coaxed Michael to drink a cold can of vanilla ENSURE--a nutritional diet-aid drink. This was not his idea of gourmet dining. He gave me that notorious dead-pan stare of his, but no complaint.

The following day, the food was worse. She said that she lacked time to undertake laundry (I had done it the day before) and that it was too hot to shop. She played the "move the spices in the cupboard" game until it was time for her to leave. I was getting desperate. Within another week I must return home, to prepare for school commencement. Michael had to be well "set up" before I could consider leaving. By the third day, things had degenerated completely. She began to argue when I itemized her responsibilities. These included the preparation of Michael's meals, laundry, and some grocery shopping. She was particularly polite and solicitous to Michael. Either I irritated her because I expected too much of her, or because she feared being discovered incapable. When I try to recapitulate those communication difficulties, it is obvious that my own tense requests did not allay terse responses.

I gave up and called the organization which had sent this home maker, explained the situation, and she was changed the following morning. However, she shouted in fury a great deal before she departed, and neither Michael nor I had appreciated her defensive reaction. It had been an unnerving experience, witnessing the lack of communication capacities and the incompetencies of this individual. The strain of Michael's illness was sufficiently draining, without the added complication of someone with poor interpersonal skills. Top quality home care and a positive atmosphere were essential components of a support system which would be conducive to Mike's rehabilitation.

Michael and I were thrilled when the next home maker worked out well. She was gentle, slow-moving but thorough, and did not think that the assigned tasks were too menial. She would have won no awards for her cooking skills, either, but Michael was able to swallow most items. An inspecting military officer would have found fault with her cleaning methods but, since I didn't own the compulsory pair of white gloves, I closed my eyes to the inconsequential. Essentially, she relaxed Michael and they chatted happily together. He looked forward to her arrival each day. She stayed with him for about six weeks also, initially five days a week, and later every second day, until the last week she was only present two days.

Michael, by then, could fetch some groceries himself from the corner, and prepare his own meals. For two weeks we had "meals on wheels" delivered, but he found the food unappealing. His mediocre appetite and nausea worked against him. Because he slept fourteen to sixteen hours, he also resented being awakened for unpalatable meals. He ordered foods delivered occasionally, and his friends delighted in taking him out to eat. Once he was no longer incontinent, the laundry awaited my visits. Dry cleaning was no problem, either. Items could be cleaned and pressed, around the corner, in a few hours.

NOT A TOTAL WASTE

One difficult undertaking was the relocation of Penny to an apartment of her own. Michael no longer wished to share the apartment. He had accepted the fatal nature of his illness, and that his health would eventually become more precarious. He still hoped for another year or two of life. The dream for a miracle cure never left our thoughts. His discomfort about asking her, once more, to hunt for an alternative living accommodation was apparent. He insisted that I speak with Penny.

Up until his illness, I had stayed at hotels in Toronto whenever I visited. I would have felt uncomfortable staying with Michael and Penny, because I wished to avoid imposing. This irritated Michael, since he knew that Toronto hotels were fairly expensive and we were assisting him financially. However, Penny's parents and brother frequently stayed for evenings or week-end visits at the apartment. Michael enjoyed Penny's family and, since I had met them, I could certainly see why. Like Penny, they were friendly, charming and well-travelled. Michael felt uncertain about the state of his health, not knowing when he would be well or very sick. He yearned for the sanctity of his own, private domain.

The situation was not a pleasant one to broach. Three months prior to Michael's illness, he had asked Penny to hunt for a new place. His illness had forced his resignation from his teaching career and placed him on disability for the past half year. He was definitely dealing with an uncertain future, healthwise. Penny had not searched for a new location. At the hospital, after Michael's brain biopsy, Corey and Ted had asked her if she had located a new apartment, and she had stated,

"It's not my responsibility to find one. That's my friends' job."

Corey said, "Are you telling us that you haven't even tried to find a new place to live?"

She became vexed and left early. Now, with arrangements finalized for Michael's nurse and home maker, it was essential to campaign for Michael's privacy. Perhaps because I was over-tired, I did not voice the urgency of this request rationally. It's also feasible that my intent to protect Michael's health, at any cost, was viewed as neurotic. No doubt Penny was masking considerable pain over Michael's impending death. They had been friends for a long time. Penny's reaction was indignation. She expressed a fondness for Michael and the inexpensive, convenient living arrangements. Michael was too ill to cope with any emotional discomfort and refused to discuss the situation any further.

Lucy and Therese intervened with an offer to assist in Penny's move. They agreed that Michael's health demanded privacy and additional space to provide for the possibility of a full-time nurse. Time was running out for Michael, even though we preferred to ignore that fact. He stipulated that he did not want either Penny, or her family, to witness his continuing health deterioration. Nevertheless, moving out was too painful a decision for Penny. She avoided it as long as possible. Therese and Lucy found three apartments available, but these did not answer Penny's requirements. As a temporary measure, she moved in with Therese and Lucy, instead.

Anna drove over from Hamilton and assisted Penny in her packing. The boxes were stored in the front room, piled to the ceiling. Penny had previously planned to visit with her sister in Edmonton, so Therese and Lucy obligingly moved her belongings to their apartment the second week-end in September. Within six months, Lucy and Therese found Penny new accommodation, redecorated it to her liking, and transferred her furniture. It has been disclosed that Penny has become thoroughly contented in her own apartment. The move was at too great a price, however. She had left with mingled feelings of anger and a sense of unworthy treatment. Michael expressed more disappointment than injury from the situation. It's hard to say who lost most from that inextricable experience, but the grave illness of a good friend or loved one has a profound effect upon everyone involved.

CHAPTER THREE

Communication problems are not unusual, when dealing with a life-threatening illness. Problems which existed before are often magnified. It should not have surprised me to discover that my own marriage was jeopardized, indirectly due to Michael's sickness. Bruce and I had been married for nearly forty years, but the relationship became increasingly dysfunctional as Michael's prognosis became apparent. The strain between us escalated. In struggling to come to grips with the terminal illness of our only son, my husband and I were not effective in sharing our agony. Sometimes we could talk together about the changing stages of the disease. More often, we were totally frustrated in trying to comprehend what was happening to Michael, and the impact of his illness upon our own relationship.

Mood swings turned us upside down. We optimistically clung to our hopes for Michael's survival, or we became deeply depressed because he would die. The grief cycle overwhelmed us both. Our individual coping mechanisms were acquired skills, taught from our own childhood. Withdrawal or anger appeared to be Bruce's methods. He loved Michael too, but was ineffectual in expressing emotion. Bruce's discomfort in offering affection was not unique to the particular situation of Michael's illness. He was a quiet, inscrutable individual who bottled up his fears, his anxieties, his rages, until he lashed out in violence. He was incapable of overtly showing his feelings. He did not exhibit anger or affection readily.

His British mother had often bragged to me that she had brought her son up "by the book". She had read somewhere that she should not show him any overt display of love or emotional attachment up until the age of seven. She often talked of breastfeeding him only at specific times of the day, to avoid producing a spoiled or pampered child. He was not picked up or cuddled, if he cried. She believed that this regimen would produce a strong, silent, stoic man. I have to admit that when he courted me, I had regarded his dignified reserve and steady calmness attractive. I had interpreted his silence as strength, and anticipated a solid relationship. Since mine had been an abusive and rejecting family, I longed for the stability and security which I had been denied.

Too often in any marriage, both parties come together encumbered with the emotional burdens of their upbringings. These make the marriage more complicated, but not entirely impossible. Bruce and I had experienced our share of misunderstandings, but pulled together as a team when things got rough. Our inherent shyness and reticence caused us some awkwardness. Society expected women to socialize, so I was more talkative. Bruce's silent isolation became a barrier.

I understood loneliness. When Anna and Michael were toddlers, an aggressive, loud-mouthed next-door neighbour hollered across the fence one hot August morning,

"Hey, Maria, are you the Virgin Mary?"
"Why? What does that mean?" I felt baffled.
"Well, where's Bruce? How come you're painting that fence by yourself? Doesn't he ever help you? Did you have those two kids completely by yourself?"

His attack both embarrassed and provoked me. It was humiliating that outsiders realized that I was predominantly responsible for rearing the youngsters. I wished that Bruce could have enjoyed and played with them more. Raising the children was a demanding job, but frequently fulfilling. We had chosen to have the children early in our marriage. We owned little furniture, a modest home, and a dilapidated car, but the children offered us much delight.

Since Anna and Michael had been born only fifteen months apart, and we were a nucleated family with a limited network of

NOT A TOTAL WASTE

friends, caring for the children sometimes got frantic for me. They were not physically strong babies, and the pressures of fevers and childhood illnesses were all mine. Bruce was unaware that the workload was unbalanced. He fed Anna her bedtime bottle, since I was feeding Michael, but did not offer extra help. Perhaps I should have told him that I needed his assistance. I had been raised with the necessity to help other family members, and he had been raised with housekeepers. Happily, he always took care of the garbage, cut the lawn, shovelled snow, and helped fetch the groceries. However, he blithely assumed that everything else would fall into place, as if by magic.

We purchased our first small home when the children were infants, and invested our time in the children and the house. There was neither time nor interest in a social life. Bruce worked, and I was the homemaker. After experiencing the loss of three additional infants through stillbirth and miscarriages, I became determined to finish my education. Bruce had graduated through scholarships as a Professional Engineer. It had made me uncomfortable that I had not completed high school, since I had worked in industry before our marriage. I thought that I'd gain confidence in being able to provide for the children, should that be necessary. I also hoped to earn additional funds to enrich our lives. I needed to be among other people, to expand my personal horizons, and to prove myself capable. When I approached Bruce about my plans, he brushed them aside. Either I expressed myself inadequately, or he was not interested.

I decided to make enquiries about night school courses, and apply. My personal fears of failure were as great as my concern about actually getting to class. Since I rarely left the house without the children, and almost never left the house at night, raising the topic required real effort. Using subterfuge, I asked Bruce to babysit one evening a week while I met with various neighbourhood women. I was too bashful to explain that I was attending night school.

He seemed puzzled by my absences each Tuesday evening, but made no comment. On the third week he met me at the door upon my return. He looked me steadily in the eyes, and said,

"Who did you say you were going shopping with to-night? Was it the lady down the street?"

I regarded him cautiously and could neither nod, nor fib. He knew that I had tried to concoct a story to cover my absence. I responded evasively.

"Why? Am I late?"

"No, but you got off the bus alone. What is so heavy in this bag?" he asked, as he took my coat and purse.

I sighed, and sat down on a nearby chair.

"They're school books. I'm taking a grade thirteen course at Central."

"You are?"

"Yes. Because I want to graduate. I want to finish my education, so that I can teach."

"Why didn't you tell me that, instead of just saying you were going shopping?"

"You didn't want to hear about it. I tried."

"So each Tuesday night you've fed us, put the kids to bed, and taken the bus to school?"

"I didn't think you'd notice whether I was here or not. You just bury yourself in the newspaper, or the television."

"You should have told me. I've been wondering what the hell was going on."

"I hardly ever go out. Do you resent me going to school once a week?"

"No. It's not that. I knew that you had no money to go shopping, and you never came home with any purchases. It made no sense. I didn't know what to think."

"Well, I am also completing two courses by correspondence with the Ministry of Education. I work on them in the afternoon, when the children are having their naps. The Physics is so hard for me that I have to take it at night school, as well."

He started to laugh, shook his head in amazement, and carefully hung up my coat. With his encouragement, I graduated from high school. It was a nightmare, studying and preparing for examinations, sandwiched in between all of the duties required at home. The examinations were written in a nearby high school. It was humiliating for me to file into the gymnasium with staring adolescents and curious teachers. I was only in my late twenties, but they made me feel like ninety. I remember turning to one gawking student, and said,

NOT A TOTAL WASTE

"I hope that you studied hard for your Trigonometry, or it may take you this long to get it, too."

She turned away quickly, and I concentrated on the paper in front of me. Afterwards, she and her young boyfriend offered me a lift home in their car. When they stopped at my corner, I noticed that the babysitter had put the children outside to play. Anna and Michael stood and watched as I got out of the fancy, low-slung sports car.

"Mommy, Mommy!" they shouted and started to run towards me.
"My God, are those your kids?" the teen-agers asked.
"Yes. Aren't they beautiful?" was my reply, and I walked proudly away from their opened mouths. The children were a powerful incentive for my study efforts.

Bruce left Engineering the following summer, and began to teach Mathematics and Physics in a local secondary school. The following year he moved north to teach, and the children and I remained behind to sell the house and pack. It was another year before we joined him. I worked part-time at secretarial jobs, and two years later wrote government trade examinations which permitted me to teach on a temporary contract. At that time, the province was short of teachers. I completed teaching methodology courses during three summers in Toronto, and University courses by extension throughout the school year. Trying to study, teach and keep things going with the family was a heavy load. In retrospect, I wonder how I did it. My education was obtained on a part-time basis, as I worked and raised the children.

Certification requirements demanded that I spend three consecutive summers separated from the family, studying in Toronto. In a way, that was an asset for Bruce and the children. Anna and Michael learned to canoe, fish and enjoy the outdoors while camping with their father. Those summers provided very special memories for them, and they appreciated one another better. I missed them all so much, and questioned my own sanity in undertaking studies in the heat and loneliness of the city. I really yearned to be enjoying the summers with them.

Obtaining my education was not an easy sacrifice, and I cried into the pillow many a night from sheer frustration. I was torn by my desire to complete my education and my need to be with my family. I never mentioned the difficulties involved, but reassured them often that I loved and missed them. They certainly didn't suffer from a domineering, over-protective mother. I was kept busy just juggling work, study and home responsibilities.

Both youngsters developed into delightful, interesting and complicated adolescents. We were very proud of them. Anna became more of an extrovert, able to make friends readily. She experienced an easy, close relationship with her father. We shared an artistic creativity, mirrored in our crafts and shopping exploits. Michael's affiliation with his father matured as a respectful aloofness. They were both very much alike in their quiet, soft-spoken mannerisms. Their reticence and dignity kept them at arms length, but there was an apparent appreciation for one another's intelligence and humour. I valued Mike's measured opinion on such diverse subjects as university research, furniture arrangement, clothing purchases or the dinner menu.

Bruce took a keen interest in the different countries which Michael visited with his studies, and was proud of his linguistic and scholastic abilities. We would talk of some day visiting all of the places where Michael had lived, to see them through his eyes. Although Bruce grumbled about the cost factor, he always backed Michael's every study venture. He often stated that he could not have selected a better ambassador to represent Canada than our son. Unfortunately, because of Bruce's reserve, he never did express those thoughts to Michael.

Anna conversed more effectively with Bruce than Michael or me, but essentially we were all immersed in our studies. Teaching requires heavy marking and lesson preparations. In addition, I was cramming courses by correspondence and night school. Shared spare time evolved around homework or housework. We were all exhausted at the end of most days, and refrained from idle chatter. If we imposed upon Bruce when he didn't feel like talking, he distracted himself by day-dreaming, turned to the television or newspaper, or changed the subject to divert us. At other times he bottled up anger or sentiments, until he exploded in short bursts of rage. Like every family, we experienced disputes and disagreements.

NOT A TOTAL WASTE

A combination of work stress and exhaustion made discussions within the family strained. Frequently, Bruce sent us such confusing mixed messages, that we withdrew and allowed him privacy. When irritated at a family member, he would sigh and say, "I love you..." in a calm nearly friendly manner. However, anger was apparent by his body language, voice or facial expressions. These apparent inconsistencies made it uneasy for all of us to feel relaxed or close with one another, but we plodded along and coped from day to day.

Whenever I forced an issue to obtain a response from Bruce, I only succeeded in making the relationship testy. In futility, I urged him to identify his feelings. I would ask him," What are you feeling right now?" Feedback was provided by starting out with, "You appear to be..." Rarely, he'd respond--and then we could openly discuss his sensibilities. By talking about his emotions, and not burying his feelings all of the time, he exhibited an awareness that his responses were normal or abnormal reactions. I suppose that we handled the good and bad patches which every family experiences, in the best way that we could. Probably the most important thing was that we both wanted the marriage to work, and loved our children.

However, when it came time for me to inform Bruce of Michael's homosexuality, as I had promised Michael I would, Bruce's reaction surprised me. I feared that he would react with frustration and bitterness. In contrast, I saw his eyes fill with concern and helplessness. Our initial feelings of anger, fear and compassion which Michael's lifestyle fostered in each of us, later changed to powerful needs for love, forgiveness and protection.

Bruce agreed that Michael's life would be more difficult due to the ignorance of society, regarding his sexual preferences. Little did we know then, that Michael would be regarded by some individuals as one of society's lepers. Persecution of homosexuals as a "third sex", or "sexual invert" was not novel. However, we knew nothing of the "gay plague" at that time, or our concerns would have multiplied.

The information that Michael had tested HIV positive was never volunteered to Bruce. I tried a few times to tell him, but each time my throat filled with emotion, and I changed the topic. How can you explain something like that easily, when your stomach feels as if one thousand knives are being pushed in and twisted? One night while watching some television footage related to the AIDS epidemic, Bruce turned to me and asked,

"You don't suppose that Michael could have that disease, do you?"
"Why?"
"Well, he is gay. He seems pinched and drawn. His life style would be a precursor for that infection, wouldn't it?"
"Bruce, he has tested HIV positive. He is carrying the virus in his blood."
"He has it? You're telling me that he has it?"

I tried hard to compose myself by holding onto the arms of the chair to gain false courage. My mind seemed to draw a blank and I began to tremble.

"Michael tells me that people can remain healthy for many years with the virus."
"You're saying that he is already infected. Does he have this AIDS they talked about?" His voice became loud and threatening.
"Please, Bruce, wait. Don't shout at me. We don't know if infection with the HIV virus automatically leads to AIDS."
"Oh, Christ...that poor little bugger. He's blown himself up. He's destroyed his life. He's done this to himself."
"Michael doesn't have to die. Maybe the amount of virus, and the additional infections of other viruses, influence how fast it turns to AIDS. There's world-wide research going on..."
"Oh, no. Oh, no."
"Stop it. Listen. We have to have some hope. Look at the stats, Bruce. Half of the individuals with HIV don't develop AIDS until ten years of getting the infection in the first place. Another quarter of them experience AIDS-related sicknesses. That gives us time to hope for a cure."

My mind was whirling, grasping any information that I had stored, trying to provide protective armour against the horrifying implications of this disease. Bruce's reaction caused me so much upheaval that I withdrew, and responded like an automation.

NOT A TOTAL WASTE

"There is no relief from this. He's ruined his life. It's his own damn fault. That bastard. He chose his life style. He's going to die." His face was flushed with anger, and his jaw was set. He glared back at me.

"You can't count him out yet. You don't know anything for certain. You can't be sure."

"He's going to get sicker and sicker. He'll drain us financially, just as he has with his education. He'll die. Just let him go. Let him die."

I stared at him. He was raging because of fear. This was our only son, and he knew that we could lose him to this disease. He was shouting because he was upset, not because he didn't love Michael. He was not alone in his torment.

"Look, what the hell do you think I am? An android? I've got feelings. I'm scared too. But maybe Mike can fight this. We have to think positively, and pray to God for a cure." I sat facing him, trembling as tears coursed down my face.

Bruce stared at me and his face clouded in rage. He threw the newspaper down, swore and went down the hall to the bathroom. The door slammed. End of conversation.

Once Michael's brief teaching career was ended, Bruce's anger grew into an irritable discontent. Fear and pain affect each family member differently, and our agony was profound. We each had our own deep well of misery to draw upon; our aches were close to the bone. The problems which we had previously experienced in sharing our hurts, reappeared. Bruce offered little solace. Loud words and accusations got us nowhere. We drifted apart further and further, at a time when we most needed to cling together. We survived by blunting our emotions. Speech was restrained and perfunctory.

Michael was aware that all was not peaceful at home. He had grown up in that environment, and had often wondered aloud whether or not the marriage was salvageable. Unfortunately, his illness served as both a catalyst and a scapegoat for all of our previous communication difficulties. Michael's sickness had not been a logical or predictable event in our lives. Our inability to control the dimensions of Michael's mortality baffled us. We tried to face the fact that all life is vulnerable and that survival is often compromised. We recognized that, in fact, we are ALL dying. But ALL was still out there, somewhere--a vague, uncertain, grey area-- not here, close to our hearts, part of our very souls. We developed a conscious need to overprotect everyone that we loved. However, people can't survive huddled in glass cages, either.

Bruce asserted himself as a death-denying father. He was furious that a fragile virus could imperceptibly enter Michael's body and destroy his immune system functions. Bruce's fears of the alienation and disaffection which our son could suffer because of society's homophobia, were mirrored within our marriage relationships. The pressure from many people within our community, and their view of gays, also made things more complicated. Homosexuality was viewed as evil and disgusting. The disease was considered as "just deserts" for a lifestyle different from the norm. AIDS patients should suffer banishment or separation from their loved ones, as punishment. Crushing judgments and imposed shame took a toll on our marriage. The lack of integration of homosexual persons into the mainstream of life, the lack of any guarantees of their personal rights and dignities frustrated us, as well. We felt understandable outrage at the discrimination against AIDS patients by society. Their treatment was unconscionable. Society's cruelty stung like a slap in the face.

Our hearts were torn when we thought that outsiders, who did not even know Michael, would consider him as an objectionable social deviant. Snide remarks made in the staff room about someone acting "GAY", or derogatory comments made from one student to another about someone's "FAGGY HAIR" made us freeze. One afternoon a male teacher sat next to me in the staff lunch room, discussing the reason for the transfer of his son to a different school.

"I told Blair that he would have to move to Western High School. We can't stand that physical education teacher any longer. We're uncomfortable about the way the teacher interacts with his students."

"What do you mean? He appears to be a very devoted coach; he gives so much of his spare time to each of the teams."

"That's one of the reasons. He's also not married. Why does he offer to drive them to their out-of-town games?"

NOT A TOTAL WASTE

"I guess he wants them to do well. Perhaps he wants to be there to encourage them."

"It makes Tina and me uneasy. This guy's just too damned available."

"That bothers you?"

"I think the creep is gay. It's not normal to spend so much time with students. He doesn't act feminine, or anything. But he's abnormal. I'm moving my kid to the other school."

I felt discomfort. From all appearances, it seemed that the coach was doing a superlative job. He may well have been gay, despite any lack of evidence. However, instead of appreciation for the long hours he gave in coaching, this parent offered criticism. Some people were quick to condemn, because of paranoia. I wondered about Michael, and how he would handle scorn and alienation. I kept my fears to myself, but I was despondent.

However, Michael's own indomitable will to survive amazed us both. He faced his illness head-on, unflinching, pushing one foot ahead of the other. He hoped to beat the odds, trying always for control of the disease, while he awaited the discovery of a cure. Even though we feared that the societal stigmatization surrounding AIDS could dehumanize and set Michael apart, his courage and strong will did not abate.

This same strength of purpose was obvious near the end of Michael's life. Three days before he died, he obtained Soloflex body-building equipment. He had intended it to be set up in his front room, so that he could exercise his wasted body back to health. In addition, he had ordered specific vitamins, which were not opened before his death. These had been touted as capable of restoring both physical vigor and abundant hair growth. Despite his waning strength, he had been persistently determined to make a come-back, and survive. His courage--to the very end of his life-- served as a beacon, for us to follow.

Michael seldom expressed his own apprehensions and tensions related to his disease. He explained to his grandmother that he had leukemia. If I felt distrust when someone asked me what was wrong with him, I would also use the same excuse. We hated to hide the truth. Certainly, Mike had cancerous lesions in his bowel, lungs, esophagus and larynx. We found it easier to withdraw, turtle-like, into our own protective shells when threatened by curious interrogations. We were in such pain knowing that we could lose Michael that we craved acceptance, not disapproval. There were always people who delighted in picking away at our emotional scabs. We were circumspect in our disclosures and guarded our privacy carefully. We yearned to express openly the type of emotional turmoil we were experiencing. By sharing that hell, it might have been easier to cope.

I flew down to Toronto once a month, at that time, to be with Michael. There were conferences to attend, or other reasons for my visits. Spare time was spent visiting with Anna in Hamilton, and Michael. Bruce's resentment regarding my time spent away from home was related to his anger at Michael's disease. One evening in February, Michael and I were perched on his bed, watching television. He did not turn his face to look at me, but watched the flickering screen as he asked,

"Have you explained to father about my AIDS yet, Ma?"
"Yes, Mike. He knows that you're taking AZT now."
"How does he feel about that?"
"As upset as I am. He's scared, too."
"How are things with you and father? Any better?"
"Oh Mike, you know how things can develop. He's pretty mean-tempered when he's upset."
"He hasn't hurt you?"
"Not physically, but often emotionally. It's part of the game. I guess we're good at hurting each other."
"You don't have to tolerate that kind of strain, Mom. You could always live and work down here. With your qualifications, you wouldn't have any problem locating something else."
"I just don't have the stamina to make any decisions, right now, son." I stretched and sighed. Suddenly, I felt limp with exhaustion. Michael seemed to choke, and then cleared his throat. He continued to stare at the screen, and then asked,
"If not the stamina--do you have the inclination?"
"I don't know, Michael. Father and I have been through lots of rough times in our lives. He has plenty of good qualities, too. I'm not rushing towards any thoughts of separation. I'm not thinking of leaving."
"I know he has merits, Mom. I love Dad, too. But I hate to see you sad and unhappy. I suppose I just want you to experience some

nirvana. You should be surrounded with people who love you and care about you. Discard what doesn't matter."

"That's what you do, isn't it Michael? There are just so many things going on, right now. Mostly, I'm just tired. Don't worry about that situation. Neither of us can fix it right now. I'm sure we're going to make it."

"I could buy a condo, here. I've been watching the real estate section of the cable TV. Many of the apartments only require a small down-payment, since real estate has gone so badly."

"They're still very expensive, Mike. You don't have that kind of cash..."

My thoughts were rushing in different ways again. I didn't realize that he had been so worried about me that he had surveyed the potential purchase of an apartment. He had meager finances, and we were helping to defray his rent, medication, and food costs.

"We could rent it out. A loan wouldn't be difficult for you to obtain. David thinks that it is an excellent time to purchase property. It's a smart investment. Prices on downtown condominiums have been slashed."

"Michael, let's not rush into anything like that. How could you handle the pressure? You don't need that kind of stress."

"I said, I could rent it out, through an agency. And I could get a car. I've kept my license up to date, in case. You wouldn't have to use the subway after dark. My bike is too difficult for me, now, anyhow."

"That's an idea. You could drive a car, to get around the city easier. Michael, we could lease you one."

"I've been giving it some thought. But Mom, if you don't want to think of a condo now, you can come and live with me. You could rearrange the front room. You can come here any time, whenever you want. You know that, Mom. And you could keep living here, after I am dead."

I froze. "After I am dead", he'd said. I did not respond to that statement, because I was blinded by tears that I must not shed. Michael did not need more agitation than he felt already. I could not cry and perturb him further. He had been seriously worried about his father and me. I blinked away the tears and did not sniffle. Each time he stated that he would die, I cringed inside. I wanted to pretend it would never happen. I hated to hear Michael talk of his impending death.

The previous November, his health had begun to show early signs of deterioration. I had been in Toronto, and we had gone to The Parrot for dinner. He had sat across the table from me, and held my hand tightly in his frail one. He remarked,

"Mom, I think I can make it through the rest of this winter, and maybe the summer, if I'm lucky. You know how it is. I'm just living on borrowed time."
"Your blood count is down? The doctor said it was this bad? Isn't there some other way?" I could feel mounting panic overwhelming me, but I tried to focus on his answers.

"There's nothing out there to help, Mom. It's just a matter of months, probably. But listen to the music, Mom. Listen. Remember what it says. And that I love you, very much."

The background music playing in that restaurant had been NON, JE NE REGRETTE RIEN, and it was being sung by France's little sparrow, Edith Piaf. I cannot control the stirring of sentiment whenever I hear it. The prayed-for magic bullet which would destroy the virus killing my son, and other mother's children, had not been developed. As the actor in the film LONGTIME COMPANION had said, "If only that time would come..."

Now in late February we sat, watching television, and he was concerned about his parents and his impending death. It seemed as though he wanted to take care of things, to fix everything, before he died. He knew that we had all experienced problems in communicating with his taciturn father. It must have hurt him that his father did not visit, nor phone, nor write. It was a few moments before I reached over and patted his hand. I said, calmly,

"Mike, don't worry about your father and me. I promise you that I will not make any rash decisions. Things will settle into place. It's all part of my own upbringing, too, Mike. You know...we marry, have babies, grow old and we die. Divorce has never really been a positive alternative. I'll give it at least a year after your death. Okay? And then father will probably be retiring, and he should mellow, right? Mike, it's only natural that we're upset right now. We both love you, and we're worried about you. Our emotions impact upon every aspect of our lives. It's bound to affect the entire nutty marriage."

NOT A TOTAL WASTE 93

"Okay, Mom."
"You know your father well. He's a good man. Anna says that there are lots worse out there. He does love us, you know."
"Yeh, in his own weird way. I know that."
"Anna says that we don't always notice it. He rarely says it."
"She's right."
"We're working at it, dear. Please don't worry."
"All right. But if things get drastic, you can always come here. At any time, for however long you want."
"Thanks, Michael."

I swallowed hard, and kept pretending to watch the television film with Michael. In a few moments he cleared his throat and turned towards me. Calmly, he adjusted his blanket which covered him and asked,

"Mom, what about Jenni's violin lessons?"
"I think she is taking piano keyboarding right now, with the intention of getting back to the violin in the fall."
"She's good at the violin, isn't she?"
"Her instructor said that Jenni was headed for professional training."
"I'd give up eating if it would pay for her lessons."
I winced. "That's the last thing that we want, Mike."
"Is Sean still working on his sketching?"
"Yes. You haven't seen his art lately. It's not bad. He's a good student, a great athlete, loves music, and has now shown skills in art. Wonder who he reminds me of..."
"Hmmm. Must be Father," he responded, with mischief sparkling in his eyes.
"Sure. Anyhow, Michael, relax about the costs for the lessons. It's no problem. I can cover that. Just take it easy. Things will fall into place. With everything, including Father. Say, do you remember what the pediatrician said to you when you were about six years old? You had asked him why he was so grumpy. He explained that the older a person gets, the more he gets like himself--more irritable or more enjoyable."
"Hmph! Does that portend well for Father? I wonder. Well, you won't have to surmise about how much I'll change in my old age, Ma. Guess I'll stay forever young and charming." He snorted, and shook his head.

"You will to those who love you, Mike. Forever young and charming."

He settled back against the pillows, and quietly watched the film.

CHAPTER FOUR

Memories of those visits with Michael continue to haunt me. I feel his presence close to me, and I hear his voice as if he is just around the corner. Different things will trigger those thoughts. Sometimes it will be smelling the scent of Javex which I used so often to disinfect Michael's apartment, seeing Michael's silk shirt that now hangs in my closet, hearing the melody of, "I Just Called, To Say I Love You" from my music box, or even observing a can of baked brown beans on a grocery shelf.

When I sort through my own clothes closet, I regard many outfits which were worn on particular festive or distressing occasions, shared with Michael. It does not matter where I am, or what I am doing. I am powerless to stop the impact of those images. They cannot be instantly intellectualized away. They encompass me, whirl about me, and carry me to another time and place, without my control.

In my mind's eye I see Michael as a happy, effervescent youngster, rushing home from school with his school work clutched tightly in his hand, talking excitedly about how high the rain water level has reached on his new boots. I see him patiently selecting various coloured patches for us to sew on the machine to produce his bedcovering. Next, he sits absorbed at the kitchen table, enclosing tiny green-glass emeralds within a broach for my surprise. Or I see him seriously explaining that I must not cry before he leaves on the plane. It will take him to live in Brazil for a full year, and he will not write home if I make a scene at the airport. I am to be brave and smile, or else.

In retrospect, I see him walking across the stage at graduation, accepting his accolades with a grin and wink for me. The black and gold gown is stretched tightly over his broad shoulders, and his blond hair is a golden helmet under the bright lights. These, and many other images, converge upon me during quiet and busy times. My emotions become raw and frayed, and I am vulnerable. I want to reach out to touch him, to tell him how much I love him, but time has become an unreliable commodity. Just as suddenly the apparitions have vanished, and reality is all that I hold in my hands.

Michael's concern for the stability of our marriage was not unfounded. Many marriages and friendships have dissolved under the death-related stress of caring for a child with AIDS. Once the diagnosis has been confirmed, lives are modifed drastically. Physical and emotional reactions have frequently compromised the relationships of the afflicted person, as well as those individuals who are most closely related to him. Initial troubles within the family unit, prior to the discovery of homosexuality and an AIDS infection, have caused the disclosure to rip a family apart. Loved ones are often stunned and shocked, unwilling to accept such tragic news.

Telling Anna about Michael's homosexuality and HIV status had not been as difficult as I had assumed. Perhaps, since she had been close to Michael as they grew up, it was not a value judgement that concerned her. She was, however, concerned by the news, and fearful of repercussions for her family.

"Anna, you realize that Michael is homosexual, don't you?"
"Well, I guess I've always wondered. The closest female relationship he ever had was with Sherry, and somehow that never developed. We all loved Sherry so much, that I expected more than a good companionship. He missed her when she returned to New Zealand. I thought that they'd meet again, and maybe get married. I was curious also when the marriage he spoke of with Lucy did not come to fruition. How did this happen to Mike, Mom? What made him gay?"

NOT A TOTAL WASTE

"Oh, Anna, there have been some debunked myths. No-one knows for sure. The old idea of the dominating mother and the disinterested father has been refuted. Any mother will instinctively over-protect her son if he is rejected by a tight-lipped or undemonstrative father. The most recent studies have verified that it is likely a genetic trait. Homosexuals don't select their lifestyle. They are born that way."

"Then do they turn the blame back onto the mother, because her body nourished the fetus as it developed within her womb?"

"Maybe at one time, they did. But if you've noticed the most recent magazine articles stipulate that the health of both parents can influence the genetic development of the embryo, so that no one person is blamed. The husband's health is just as influential in producing a healthy baby. Society has generally recognized the obvious link between mother and child, but had previously disregarded male reproductive system hazards. If the husband is a heavy smoker, or if he works with toxic chemicals, it could affect his sperm. Those are recognized risks."

"So therefore, if homosexuality is inherited, it can be transferred from either the egg or the sperm. You know Mom, I remember reading that in some cultures homosexuals are actually revered, and treated as unique or special. They are considered capable of advising both male and female members of their society."

"It makes sense. Because of the AIDS deaths, some scientists had done some related brain studies. Male and females have a different spatial capacity between the left and right hemispheres of the brain. For some reason females are able to transfer thoughts more readily from their left to their right brain. Apparently, the homosexual male's brain was ascertained to be more similar in shape to the female brain. This may not have been verified. It could just be one person's opinion."

"Sounds discriminatory to me."

"You may be right about that. I guess the main thing that the newest research states is that the homosexual was born in the way that he develops. He did not determine his differences. Sexuality is genetic. So what. I wouldn't want Michael any different than he is, would you?"

"No, Mom. We all love him, and wouldn't want him changed. There would be a big, empty hole in our lives without him."

"That's something else that we may have to contend with, dear. Has he told you that he is HIV positive?"

"What does that mean? Do you mean that he can get AIDS? Or has he got that now? How long has this been going on? How much time does he have left? Why didn't he tell me?"

Her face was ashen in colour, yet her cheeks were brightly flushed. She belted out question after question, as I sat immobile. It had been so hard to initiate this topic that I couldn't immediately answer her questions. We searched each other's eyes, hoping to find a solution to the anguish of potential loss.

When we had finished talking about the full cruel implications of Michael's illness, Anna felt uncomfortable about disclosing it to Sean and Jenni. Although Anna did share this information with Bernie, her husband, he was not able to provide much positive reinforcement for her. Since their own marriage, Bernie had experienced the deaths of his adopted parents from cancer. He and Anna had successfully searched for his birth parents. After building an enviable, loving relationship with his father, he had recently lost him to cancer, as well. He needed to protect himself against dealing with additional death effects, wherever possible. He was fond of Mike, too, and would find it difficult to accept his terminal illness.

Because she requested it, we went along with the charade that Michael was suffering from leukemia. This provided an alternative explanation for the children. It was not until a year after Michael's death that I comprehended how carefully Anna had detailed the full implications of his AIDS-related death to Sean and Jenni. During a televised AIDS benefit program in July of 1992, Sean cleverly explained to Jenni the reasons for safe sex and the purpose for protecting themselves against a tortuous death, such as their uncle Michael had experienced. After we had discussed it together, they understood that by the year 2000 the number of infected persons worldwide could reach over 100 million--three times earlier estimated totals. They learned that women around the world account for 50 percent of HIV infections, and that showed a 25% increase from the previous year. When we discussed the geographical impact of the disease, they understood that Asia would lead the world in HIV infections by the beginning of the next century. Because of their youth, it was important for Jenni and Sean to realize that this disease would be a continuing crisis throughout their adolescence. As it touched newborns, hemophiliacs, straight men and their unsuspecting wives, it would no longer be considered merely a junkie's curse or a gay disease.

NOT A TOTAL WASTE

Bruce and I were well aware that due to the ignorance of rednecks and zealots, the publicity of Michael's illness could affect our own teaching careers. We could not possibly contaminate our students, but many people are decidedly illiterate regarding the related facts of the disease. Trying to sort out personal feelings of guilt, betrayal, and heightened emotions took time. Like Michael, what his loved ones required was empathy and compassion, not public censure. Real family values were about love, respect and caring. Homosexuality did not negate those concepts. Our loyal friends provided loving support throughout our time of crisis.

The marriage still encountered a few stumbling blocks. As Michael's health continued to decline, increased stress was indicated by Bruce's reactions. I was packing my overnight bag, on an October Friday morning, prior to leaving for school. Shirley, a dear friend, had promised to drive me to the airport. Bruce was busily shaving in the bathroom, when I interrupted him to get my toothpaste and toothbrush.

"You're off again, eh?" He had spoken sharply. I cringed, and replied as softly as I could.
"Yes. I reminded you about that, last night."
"Why don't you just move in with that little bugger."
"Pardon?"
"You're down there all the time. Why don't you just stay and not bother to come back at all."
"Bruce, stop this. Don't say something that you'll regret later. You're going to break something that can't be mended." My stomach was in knots. I felt shocked and bewildered.
"I'm fed up with all of this. Look at you. You're haggard, and you still keep pushing yourself. Why the hell don't you just tell him to take care of himself? Or better yet, just die and get it over with."

I retreated from him, and returned to my packing. My eyes burned with tears. DAMN you, Bruce. DAMN, DAMN, DAMN. Can't you care about Michael now, when he needs our support so earnestly? I made a futile mess of packing. I was completely worn out, confused and indignant at Bruce's cruel remarks.

Bruce strolled into the bedroom and observed my chaos. His bath towel was wrapped around his lean, muscular body. He crossed his arms and stared at me defiantly. When I look back at that terrible time, it is obvious that his worry over Michael's declining health was increased by his regard for my exhaustion.

"How long do you think that this is going to continue? How long do you expect that little leech to live?"
"Stop it--Stop It--STOP IT. Don't hurt me like this. For God's sake Bruce, he's our only son. He's dying. He deserves all of the help that we can give him. Why are you upsetting me, now? You know that he has so little time left!"

The tears came easily now, cascading down my cheeks and forming little rivulets into the corners of my mouth. I licked away the salty taste and chewed on the corner of my lip. My chest heaved with sobs that wanted to burst out. My thoughts were confused and disoriented.

"Why can't you just stay home. Let him manage on his own. We've poured money out. You've arranged everything for him. Leave him be. Get some rest and spend some time with me."

I turned my back on him and groped for nylons, makeup and hairbrush to put inside the bag. I could not respond. He didn't speak for a minute, and then he icily stated,

"While you're down there, get a blood test."
I whirled around, and stared at him in amazement.
"What the hell are you saying? What are you trying to insinuate? Stop this. Why can't you acquire some of Michael's kindness and gentle manners?"
"He can afford to be gentle. What the hell else does he do all day?"
"Why are you acting like this? WHY? You don't give a damn about me or Michael. You probably never did."

I stood very still, grasping the side of the suitcase for strength. I could not understand why this attack had started. It was so savage, and it ripped right through me.

"We've wasted enough cash on him. Let him die."
"He loves you, Bruce. But just listen to you. You're letting him down, and me too. You haven't seen or spoken to him in two years. You fly down to see your mother, in the same bloody

NOT A TOTAL WASTE 101

city...but you won't go to Michael, or write him, or phone him. You ignored your father in the same way when he died of cancer. Anna, Michael, and I visited your father, but you wouldn't. You're a mean bastard. You know that Michael's dying...DYING. Do you hear me?''

''You hysterical bitch.''

''I am NOT hysterical. I'm damned angry. It takes strength to be kind. You have none.''

We stared at each other. Bruce was standing rigidly still and I was quivering. His phobia related to illness or death was hard to accept. He suffered intensely, too. His inappropriate actions, however, negated those feelings. Sometimes, one small sentence can destroy what has taken years to build. Bruce's body gestures and grimaces spoke of searing disgust. His appearance, his stance and his words continue to haunt me. How punitive we can appear, to those we are supposed to love the most. He cocked his head to one side, measured his thoughts carefully and then said,

''You're at risk. You are the one who is looking after all of his needs. You're putting ME at risk. I'm telling you to get a blood test before you come back here.''

''Bruce, how can you be so ignorant? I take every precaution. I wear surgical rubber gloves. I wash every surface with disinfectant. I keep the place clean so that neither Michael nor I can end up with salmonella, hepatitis, or anything else.''

I was in such shock that I had rhymed this off like a grocery list. Facts were my only armour.

''What do you know? You're no bloody expert.''

''I'm his mother! I'm not touching Mike's contaminated blood or seminal fluids. We're not sharing needles, or exchanging blood transfusions. You don't get AIDS through casual social contact. What the hell is your problem?''

''If you know so damn much, then stay down there with him. I can do without you.''

''I guess that you can. I don't understand you. If I eat from Michael's plate, I won't get AIDS. If a mosquito bites him, I'm not going to catch it. Insects don't carry this virus. If they did, you'd have lots of children and old people with the disease. GROW UP!''

"What makes you think that you know it all? A mosquito can carry malaria."
"Yeh, and a tick can harbour Lyme's disease. A flea carried the bubonic plague. What next?"
"You don't know anything for certain. Maybe bed bugs can carry hepatitis. Or even AIDS. Do you hear me? You just don't KNOW. You could carry that damn disease back here and give it to me. Do what I told you."

He stood with his hands on his hips, and curled his lips into a sneer. He turned on his heel, stormed out of the room, and slammed the door. The door reverberated with his wooden swearing, and I sat shaking on the edge of the bed. My ulcerated stomach cramped, and my head ached from the back of my neck to my temples.

I tried to relieve the stress by rolling my head around in circles a few times to stretch the neck muscles. I dropped my lower jaw, and wiggled it to relax the tension on my chin. Slowly, I rotated my shoulders around and around, and squeezed them as high as I could. I released them, and tried to let my hands go limp, and curled my fingers. Gently, I closed my eyes and kept my breathing steady. I felt a bit better, but thoroughly exhausted.

What had started all this? Was it my fault? Why was Bruce so paranoid? He continued to sleep in the spare bedroom, on the pretext that his heavy locomotive-noise snoring would keep me from my needed rest. Obviously, he was terrified that I would give him AIDS. Because I had taken every precaution, I felt confident that I had not exposed myself to any danger. Still, I feared being tested. I couldn't face that reality, yet. A lump of anger sat hard and firm in the pit of my stomach. I would not be placated.

CHAPTER FIVE

On August 23rd I kissed Michael good-bye, on his cheek. I prayed that he'd be much stronger on my next visit, and returned to prepare for the new school year. My habit had been to telephone him every second day, and if he had sounded ill or tired, the very next day. Ma Bell would have been thrilled to know that sometimes, I called him twice during the same day. When he ran a fever or was weakened from dehydration, it was essential that I check twice. He would chuckle, remind me about the Beatles' song, and declare that he was "getting by, with a little help from my friends". His daily reassurances that he was "just fine, Ma" and his affectionate statement of, "I love you too, Mom" continually echo in my mind. As we bade farewell that week-end, he sat quietly, gathered his duvet around him regally, and regarded me fixedly. With narrowed eyes and a furrowed brow, he asked,

"Ma, you're not going to keep on calling me every day, are you?" He sounded annoyed.
"Michael, I just have to hear your voice, to know that you're okay."
"And if I don't answer the phone?"
"I'll probably flip out, and call David, or Lynda and Ryan, to check on you."
"And Ted, Corey and Kim. Mom, you have to stop phoning. Father will be having a fit about the cost."

"I can afford the phone calls, dear. I can't afford the terror, if I think you are all alone and unable to get to the phone. Your bones are so brittle now. You could easily fracture a hip, and be unable to move. You could be having a seizure, or in a coma from a fever, or starving because you can't seem to eat."

He shook his head and grinned back at me. "Well, I guess that's what mother's do...consider every worst-case scenario. It's okay if you call, Ma. Because, I guess that I won't be here...for too much longer. I like to hear your voice, too. It's all right, Ma. Don't worry."

I stopped feeling guilty about pestering him every single day at about five o'clock. I would not be satisfied to proceed with the rituals of housework and homework, until I had reassured myself that he was still there, still holding on to life through sheer determination.

Once I got back into the swing of my busy schedule, Michael seemed to be adjusting adequately. He required twelve to fourteen hours of sleep each night, which was a small improvement. However, the AZT was not helping him any longer, and by the end of August it was replaced with an experimental drug regimen, using DDI. The major side-effect for Michael seemed to be a further diminished appetite, which alarmed me. He was well aware of his reduced strength. In a letter to Sherry in New Zealand, written in early April of that year, 1990, Mike explained the impact of AIDS upon his life.

Dear Sherry,

Couldn't possibly leave you stewing down there, wondering what was going on up here, so I actually responded WITHIN TEN DAYS OF RECEIVING YOUR LETTER!!!! You know better than to expect this to happen again, of course.

Let's get the medical questions out of the way first. Yes, the T-cell count is extremely low and yes, it is an INDICATION of how far the damn thing has progressed, although it ain't necessarily so. My doctor has seen people with a T-cell count of 18 who show no signs of illness at all and are, in fact, totally asymptomatic. Sounds weird, but apparently there are other factors that affect things. I have been on AZT for a year, and according to the latest tests, it is

NOT A TOTAL WASTE

still working moderately well, although starting to wear off. When it does, I will go onto DDI, which is the next generation of drugs. By the time that is gone, there is something rather promising in Holland, etc. etc. etc. My weight has been dropping steadily--I can't seem to bring it above 143 any more. The chronic (and VERY annoying) Diarrhea is largely responsible for that. Doesn't seem to be anything I can do except spend a ton 'o money on antidiarrhetics. What fun. I have night sweats, chills, fever, and catch every little cold that comes along. I tire very easily, and need between ten to twelve hours of sleep per day. Hence the "effortless" job. However, I have NOT had ANY major illness. The mind is a bit scatterbrained, but not (much) more than (I think?) it used to be...in general, except for being so damned tired and looking so damned skinny (and between the two, looking rather haggard) I really don't feel too bad. I like loafing and listening to music, and now that summer is here (it's 32 degrees today) I can whip about a bit on the old bicycle, getting out of the house and getting exercise at the same time. Thank GOD winter is over. Mom actually broke down and cried when it snowed the second week of April (Dad had to get out the snowblower). I know how she felt.

Time for another paragraph? Re: supportive friends. I have very good, close friends who love me. I don't mention them a whole lot because you don't really know them, and I don't like to bore you with tons of dribble about people you don't know. The list includes my roommate, Penny, who puts up with an amazing amount, our mutual friend Lucy, now back from France (although off to New York for a couple of months soon), David (the dear friend who sent me to France and bought me my new CD player, and smothers me with amazing dinners), Ted (an old stand-by for ten years, extremely loyal and sweet), Corey (an advertising management type, and supportive forever), Lynda (who lives upstairs and probably has a clearer perspective on me than anyone and who I am most likely to bitch at, an ex-roomy who studied architecture with me) not to mention family. Yes, the family does know. Granny thinks I have leukemia, but otherwise everybody has a clear idea of what is going on. Mom is handling it very well. The fact that she has spent so many years training people to deal with death and dying through the palliative care workshops, and her work with the AIDS committee at home, have all helped. Enough of this topic, though. Time for another paragraph.

As mentioned earlier, ITS SUMMER! I don't know if you can have any idea how glorious those two words are for a non-winter person who has just spent the last six months cooped up inside hibernating. New Zealand has winters, but nowhere near as vile as this past one was. Everyone is more than a little delirious. I can bike to work in shorts and a T-shirt now and be WARM all at the same time. (I could have done it earlier, but probably wouldn't have been able to move my limbs for too long...)

LATER--BY A MONTH...

Well, Happy Mother's Day. I knew that this letter wouldn't end up getting to you in anything approaching a realistic time frame. Sorry.

I am watching a bit of television and reading. The weather has of course become a bit unsettled, it being early May, and the best thing to do right now is hang around the house. I quit my job, because I found I didn't have enough energy left to take care of myself (I'd come home and fall asleep, without eating, etc.) Hopefully Health and Welfare Canada will come through with a bit of money and hopefully we will get the Insurance situation straightened out. If some money does not come through, I will have to borrow again from Mom and Dad, because welfare is not enough to live on.

So, how is Timmy doing? Will you be going back to nursing, or is day care simply out of the question? Also, of course, could you stand going back to nursing? Do you really want to stay in Christchurch? I know that you wanted to be there for your family and for the kids (nice place to grow up in and all that) but any place in New Zealand really isn't that far away, and any place down there seems like a better place to grow up than, say, our Toronto.

Well, I think I've just gone through anything of any interest. Furthermore, I want to get this off to you while its still relatively current. Hope you are all well and that the financial situation is better. Take Care.

Love,

Michael.

NOT A TOTAL WASTE

When I returned to see him on September 14th, 1990 his weight was down to 130 pounds. He was not concerned about the toxicity of the DDI, but was dejected that he no longer tolerated most foods. One night on the phone he had said, "Guess what, Mom. I can't even eat fish anymore." Pork, beef and chicken had already been eliminated from his diet because of digestive difficulties. Fish had become a mainstay. He was devastated at this new deprivation.

He had avoided vegetables since his illness in June, eliminated most dairy products except milk, could not abide fruits unless in juice form, and was not at all tempted by sweet desserts. Shopping for groceries became more of a puzzle with each trip. Once he found some item which did not make him vomit, he would stay faithful to that item for days or weeks. During one such rut, cold cereals became his major meal.

That preference moved to other food groups, but his perennial favourite treat was vanilla Haagen Dazs ice cream. He would take three scoops of Haagen Dazs, one egg, one banana and a cup and a half of milk blended together smoothly. Slowly, he would sip that concoction with contentment. I tried to introduce Ensure, Ensure Plus and Boost, nutritional liquid diets, into the milkshake. My purpose was to increase the vitamins, minerals and trace elements within his diet. Michael discerned the difference in taste instantly, and forcefully regurgitated it. I had to admit defeat. Fresh strawberries were added to the mixture, without affecting his taste buds. The last three weeks of his life, this liquid and baked brown beans were his main nourishment sources. As he said to Corey, "What doesn't come right up, goes right out the other end."

However, most Saturday evenings, David would make special arrangements for dinner at various favourite restaurants in downtown Toronto. If Michael was not doing well, he would pick him up in his car. Otherwise, Michael managed to meet David independently by taxi. Whenever I was in town, I was privileged to be part of the "Saturday Night Special" treat. I have never eaten such marvellous meals, nor enjoyed such delightful companionship. I'll never forget Michael's anticipation in preparing for those exhilarating excursions.

After we had dinner with David and Kim the second week-end of October 1990, Michael felt that he was strong enough to go pub-crawling and dancing. He determined that they would drop me off first, at the apartment. I was amazed that he experienced such strength, and also felt thrilled that he wanted to get out. I said nothing to his suggestion, but looked out of the taxi window and waited for a reaction from David and Kim to his plan. At first, they were both too stunned to respond. Then they chuckled with encouragement, and waved me good-night. I grinned to myself as I let myself into the apartment. I went directly to bed, but lay there wide awake. I earnestly hoped that his evening would be a complete success.

It had been over four months since he had been "out on the town", and he definitely needed a change of scenery. The hibernation was creating despondency. Mike had labelled it "cabin fever" and "housewife-itis", meaning that he felt trapped and depressed inside the apartment. His decision to have a party time was a positive aspect, since it indicated that he felt healthy enough to re-enter his life. I heard the door open softly, Kim commented, "Good night, Mike. Do you think that you can manage by yourself?" "Sure. No problem," was Michael's weary response. I was exhilarated that he'd had a good time and grateful that he was safely home. I waited until he was in the shower, before I peeked at my watch. It was one o'clock and he was obviously very proud of this first escapade since his illness. I wanted to sing out, "Hey, good for you, Mike. Hope that you had a great time," but I played possum instead.

In the morning, Anna met me at the laundromat on the corner. She kept an eye on the driers and washers, while I went down the street to fetch bagels with cream cheese and coffee. We chatted as we folded clothes, and headed back to Michael. He was returning from the bathroom, when we entered the apartment. His delight and surprise at seeing Anna made us all feel gleeful. He had forgotten that she had offered to drive me to the airport. Ordinarily I just hired a taxi, but the trip would be a pleasure with her companionship. Michael walked towards Anna with a happy smile, but faltered and fell. As he sank down, I caught him underneath his arms, from behind. "I have you dear, just relax. I've caught you." Slowly, I lowered him to the floor. He weighed so little, but I could not hold him effectively. His forehead was bathed in perspiration, his body clammy and cold.

"Oh, Mom, what's wrong with him?"

NOT A TOTAL WASTE

"I don't know, Anna. This rascal went out partying last night."
"Michael, did you really?"
"Yeh, I guess so. I went to a few pubs, and I even danced a little bit."
"Oh-oh. Looks like you had a few too many beers, too, little brother!"
"Mike, is this just an ugly hangover?"
"I guess so, Mom. Imagine that!"

He looked both sheepish, and proud of himself, despite the resulting sickness. Anna helped me to return him to bed. Once he was in a stationary position, and the room had stopped rotating for him, I left to get some Pepto-Bismol from the corner store. I can still visualize his embarrassed but contented smile, teasing the corners of his mouth, when I left him with the medicine and spoon. He was thrilled that he had been able to get out of the apartment, even if it had been for such a brief sojourn. The painful retribution of an old-fashioned hangover was no real imposition. Because his body weight was only 130 lbs., it would have taken few beverages to produce such a profound result. The main thing was that he had avoided isolation, which he despised. He had been out dancing on a Saturday night in Toronto! Anna and I had been there, to catch him when he fell.

CHAPTER SIX

On my November 1990 visit, he had felt ambitious enough to take a walk along Queen Street on the Saturday afternoon. We toyed with tuna melts, salad and tea for lunch at the Queen Mother's, and shopped for books. It seemed to be getting dark early due to an approaching storm, so we hailed a taxi just outside of the College Street subway station. The cabbie became confused with the one-way streets in the Cabbagetown area. We paid him and decided to walk the last two blocks to Gerrard and Berkley. As we walked along chatting, I put my arm through Michael's. We were discussing the film, DRIVING MISS DAISY, when I felt Michael's body stiffen. He stopped walking. Silently, I scanned our surroundings to determine what had frightened him. Three young men walked towards us. Their heads were completely shaven, they wore black leather pants, jackets and high leather boots. Silver spikes were scattered on their apparel.

"What is it, son?"
"Just come this way, Ma. It's a shortcut."
"Okay. Let me walk beside you, dear."

Michael picked up speed that amazed me. We went through a parking lot, over a low fence, down a darkened alley, and back onto a well-lit section of the street. He turned once to see if the way was clear, and reached for my hand. We pushed forward together. We

NOT A TOTAL WASTE

got to the apartment house, out of breath and silent. His fear had been so tangible that I couldn't shake that sensation of terror, even after we had locked the door carefully and firmly behind us. Neither one of us spoke. Michael went to his bedroom and lay very still for a half hour. I pretended to read a book, but couldn't follow the plot. I wondered what would have happened, if Michael had not changed our route so rapidly. Would he have managed, if he had been alone? Would they have actually attacked him?

Previously, he had told me tales of friends who had been stalked and beaten. Michael had described how he had been punched in the side of his head as he entered a gay bar from an Edmonton street, three years previously. He was left bleeding and unconscious, and had required four days of respite in the hospital. His assailant had been a stranger. I recalled his friend Jacob explaining to us, four months before his death, that he had hired a companion to bathe and feed him. Jacob was beaten and robbed, and the hired hand was never located. During the past year a homosexual acquaintance of mine had been beaten until his legs were broken. Leslie had been abandoned on the hood of his car, unconscious. Gay bashing was not novel news. It was a nasty trend, which had already resulted in the death of a school librarian. No pleasant thoughts reassured me. Around seven o'clock, Michael reminded me that we were expected to meet David and Kim for dinner. We changed, and left to enjoy a delectable evening engagement at Biffy's Bistro.

We were both worn out from our busy day, upon our return. Michael watched KIDS IN THE HALL, and then turned off the television. We slept deeply. At 4:30 the next morning, the sounds of things falling came from the bathroom. I got up quickly and ran as fast as I could. My real fear was that Michael could have tripped and injured himself. When I got to the bathroom door, the room was empty. Listening cautiously, I pondered about the noises which had awakened me. Everything was peacefully still. Returning to the front room, I lay down and tried to sleep again. Within a matter of moments, there were louder sounds of items hitting the bathroom floor. I tiptoed down the hall, checked to ensure that Michael still slept, and headed towards the noise. Again--I saw nothing.

Frustrated, I sat on the toilet, urinated and flushed the toilet, without turning on the light. As I got up, my foot touched Michael's shaving lotion, my shampoo and bubble bath. These had been placed on the window ledge, and now lay with other items scattered on the floor. I entered the kitchen again, as I heard a type of squeaking, tearing sound. Deftly, I turned on the light. Filling the window was an outline of a man, holding a knife with a serrated six-inch blade, cutting away at the new screen. The light illuminated him well, and we stared at each other. I felt a sudden fear for Michael's safety. It did not occur to me that I might be in danger. How could I prevent this criminal from hurting Michael? He did not leave, but continued with his task of destroying the screen. I raised my voice, in order to awaken Mike.

"Michael, dial 911. There's a jerk out here, and he's cutting the screen on the kitchen window."

"Oh, shit...I've got 911, Mother."

"Michael, he won't leave. He's some kind of a nut case. I can see him very clearly, Mike. Phone Ryan and Lynda. Maybe they should know he's here, too."

"Right, Ma."

The interloper leered at me. I was terrified. My heart was beating furiously. What if he had a gun? I couldn't seem to move away from the window. I was dressed in my funny pyjamas which bore the slogan, "SAY NO TO ANIMAL TESTING". It might have been comical to watch this slow-moving episode, if I hadn't been so scared. He continued to stare at me as he took his time replacing the knife to his jacket pocket. His features were etched in my memory. His movements were careful and purposeful. He scowled at me in a menacing manner, gradually turned, and began to walk away from the window. I reached for the portable phone from the dining room book shelf.

"Michael, thank God that you answered me. He thought that I was alone. When he heard your voice, he sure didn't rush away, but he has finally gone. I'll call the police now. You just rest."

"Did you get a good look at him, Mom?"

"I sure did. He didn't know that he was dealing with an artist. I'll be able to complete a pretty good sketch of him for the police-- no problem."

Outside of Michael's window was a "GASP!", and the sound of running feet. We heard the garbage cans fly every-which-way as he fled. He had obviously walked slowly around to the side of the

NOT A TOTAL WASTE

building, and stood outside Michael's bedroom window. Michael and I stared steadily at one another.

"Sounds like you scared the hell out of him, Ma. He knows that the police will eventually trace him, with a good description."

After the police had completed their report and left, Michael asked,

"Mom, describe that guy to me, one more time?"

"He was 5'7" to 5'8" tall, medium build, dark blond shoulder-length hair, a mustache but no beard, wearing a blue plaid workshirt, jeans, no gloves, no hat, a light-brown windbreaker and a six-inch cutting blade."

"That's what I thought. It's the same guy who tried to get through my bedroom window last Saturday, at about the same time."

"What? He was here before? What did you do?"

"I didn't do anything. What could I do? I just stayed still."

"You should have called the police, Michael. They would have come. What if he'd gotten in and hurt you?"

"Ryan chased him away. When he couldn't get into the window, he leaned on my door bell for about twenty rings. If you look, you'll see that my screen has been torn completely off the window, here."

"Oh, my God. You're right. Look, I'm going upstairs to tell Lynda and Ryan right now. What if this idiot comes back and tries to break into their apartment? I'll just check with Ryan about the description. Ryan would have seen him clearly, when he chased him away."

"Good idea, Ma. Ryan travels frequently and Lynda is often alone."

I hated to bother Lynda and Ryan so early in the morning, but it seemed that this intruder was very persistent. Because of his bold mannerisms towards me, I thought that they ought to be warned. Once Ryan heard my description, he phoned the police to verify that this same trespasser had attempted to break-and-enter the previous week. Since they had been unable to apprehend him, some protective measures must be taken for Michael. In his weakened state, he could not fight off an interloper.

After notifying Bruce about what had transpired, I told Michael that I would be back after his nap. I took a taxi to Canadian Tire and purchased three window-sized security bars for the kitchen. Then, I continued to North York to a small steel-bar factory. The young owner had assured me, via the telephone, of the availability of security bars to fit the over-sized bedroom, dining room, bathroom and front room windows. I purchased white enamelled bars, ornamentally designed with detailed filigree, and white-painted screws for their attachment to the window frames.

It had been expensive to obtain these customized batch of security bars, but the cost was insignificant. Bruce urged me to take whatever precautions were necessary. His change of heart, after our last angry exchange regarding the costs of Mike's illness, was not unusual. His ranting and raving had only meant that he was angry at the disease, and its terrible toll on all of Mike's loved ones. He was miserable over the prospect of Michael's demise, and lashed out at me. Bruce asserted that Michael's safety was vital, and did not complain over the bills for the safety bars.

Half an hour after my return, Ted dropped by on his way to work. Michael had showered and shaved, and was resting in bed. When we explained to Ted about our excitement the previous night, and the newly-purchased bars, he installed the kitchen ones immediately. Unfortunately, we did not have an automatic screwdriver. By the time that he had completed his task, the palm of his right hand was reddened with blisters. How he managed to carry his serving trays at Lime Ricky's that day, we'll never know. He did not complain, but asserted that he'd come back later on to finish the job. I thanked Ted, but insisted that I'd call my son-in-law Bernie and request his help. Ted confirmed his promise, when he telephoned upon completion of his work shift.

When I contacted Anna, she explained that Bernie was out of town until the following morning, but that he could put the bars on "first thing". He also owned an electric screwdriver, which would make for an easier job. She got a babysitter to keep an eye on the children, and drove over right away. She brought Heidi, their large German Shepherd. The dog was an intelligent, R.C.M.P. obedience-trained animal, and Anna was intending to leave her with us overnight for protection. Because Michael was just recovering from toxoplasmosis, I wouldn't let her bring Heidi into the apartment. Anna felt badly, but agreed that she had not considered the

NOT A TOTAL WASTE

possible consequences of having any animal close to Michael. Her heart had been in the right place, but caution was the safest plan.

We managed fine that night without any other bars, but candidly, neither of us slept too well. Early the following morning, Anna, Bernie and Jenni installed all of the security bars. Sean was at hockey school, so he missed out on that episode. Alarms were placed on the back door, bathroom and kitchen windows. Those could be activated by pressure, and functioned with batteries.

"All done now, Mike. No-one can get into this Fort. We've got you secured."

"Thanks, Bernie. Does Mom feel better about it?"

"Yes, Mike. And so do I," answered Anna.

"I'm sorry, son. I guess you feel like you've been ensconced in a royal prison. I didn't mean to depress you. Once you've checked them out, you'll see that they're not oppressive. They're white enamelled and blend with the window frames and blinds. "

"Sure, Ma."

"Michael, don't be sarcastic. Neither Mom nor I would feel right leaving you without some kind of protection, while you're sick. Take a peek at them."

Michael raised himself on his pillows and looked at the bedroom window bars. He didn't reply to Anna, but just frowned a bit.

"Guess I'll get used to them. What do you think, Jenni? Do you think your Uncle Mike is safe, now? I felt safe enough, before."

"But Nana didn't, Uncle Mike. Now she does. You ought to see your back door. Mommy says that it looks like New York."

"What do you mean?"

"Nana and Daddy put extra locks and an alarm on the door. Mommy says they can be opened easily from the kitchen in case of fire."

"Oh, boy."

He sighed, and looked at us with that notorious stare which he usually reserved for serious offences. Anna giggled and said, "Oh Mike, don't be such a poop."

He grinned then, and everybody laughed with relief. "Barred windows do not necessarily 'a prison make', but I suppose new friends won't come visiting via the windows."

I felt more confident, leaving for the plane that afternoon. The theft of Michael's every possession would not have unnerved me, too badly. Injury to Michael would have devastated me. A few months previously, someone had sawed through the back porch bannister to steal his bicycle. That was replaced through the insurance company. No-one must get an opportunity to steal his life. Not now. Definitely, not now.

CHAPTER SEVEN

Michael and I had shared an opulant, exultant Christmas Party at David's home during the previous 1989 festive season. However, during the Christmas holiday of 1990, I was up to my ears marking essays and finalizing mid-term marks for the first half of my vacation. David had entertained for the holiday, and Michael had remained overnight at David's home during the festivities. David had promised me that he would take good care of Mike so I knew that he would not get overtired. Bruce went to Toronto for three days to visit his mother, but he neither telephoned nor visited Michael. Upon his return, I phoned Michael to see what arrangements were in place for the balance of his holiday time. He sounded depressed, without definite plans, so I departed on the morning flight.

After I had paid the limousine driver, I picked up my bag and started towards Michael's apartment. I saw an older thin man shuffling down the street about four houses away, carrying a shopping bag in each hand. He was having difficulty pushing against the wind, and was stopping frequently to adjust the heavy bags. His head was bent, and I wondered how he could handle that biting wind without the benefit of a hat. I trudged through the snow towards the steps, relieved that I did not have far to travel. Since the older gentleman was heading for the same destination, I slowed down to provide any needed assistance. After closer scrutiny, I recognized that the older man was Michael.

I unlocked the apartment door, grinned at him and moved aside to let him pass. He looked straight into my eyes with such a ragged, exposed pain that I turned away. Rather than show my emotions, I tried to lighten things up.

"Your nose is red, Santa."
"Yours would be too, if you had walked further than that limo."
"Miserable wind, and the snow doesn't want to stop."
"How was the turbulence, Mom?"
"After two cups of rum eggnog, I didn't notice."
"Not good for high cholesterol."
"No, but great for a high holiday mood. What did you buy?"
"Some milk...some beans...some Earl Grey tea...and some lemon danish for your breakfast. I wanted you to have a nice breakfast for a change."

He went into the bathroom to wash up. I sat for awhile, with the unopened bag at my feet, still in shock at the reality of how much this disease had altered Michael's appearance and stamina. He was caved in, bent over and prematurely aged. A racking cough shook his spindly body until the sputum was ejected. His condition had worsened rapidly in three weeks. He was frail and feverish. I did not offer to put away the groceries which he had purchased from the corner store. He needed what dignity he could muster, and I knew that if he got irritated with me I'd end up in tears. Despite his illness, he had shopped for me. The noise of cans placed upon shelves and milk stored in the refrigerator came down the hall. I heard the sound of the spoon against the glass as Michael mixed some DDI with water, and waited until he had drunk the medication.

"Where would you like to go to eat to-night, Mike?"
"Do you feel like Japanese?"
"That would be great. You can have your favourite sushi dish, and I'd love that shrimp soup. Do you want to rest, first?"
"No, you can call the cab, Mom."

Speaking Japanese to the waiter, Michael ordered our dinner. We sipped hot sake, a beverage made from fermented rice. The tiny entree dishes contained items which I could not identify. Michael was very distant and without an appetite. When his main meal selection arrived, he smiled wanly and made an effort to partake of

NOT A TOTAL WASTE

his favourites. I did not watch him, but busily engaged my chop sticks in the task of grasping a large breaded shrimp from the soup broth. Michael had real finesse with these cunning little sticks, but I was very awkward. Just as I nearly succeeded in getting the shrimp to my mouth, I heard Michael retch. Strangling, dry heaves shook his body forcefully. I shoved my soup bowl in front of him.

"It's okay, dear. Use this. No-one is sitting near us. Let it go."

He continued to choke and then coughed. His forehead was wet with perspiration. What should I do? What could I say? Should I just sit still and wait? I felt helpless and stupid. He looked up at me, and said,

"Sorry, Mom. I'm having trouble swallowing anything."
"Would you rather order some of this broth, dear?"
"No, Mom. It's just that...never mind."

I didn't push him for an explanation. I let it go. We sipped our jasmine tea, and he appeared to relax. When the waiter returned, I asked him to pack the balance of Michael's raw fish dinner. Michael waved his hand in irritation, but I smiled and said,

"Why not? You might like it better tomorrow."
"Don't think so, Ma. Might as well throw it out."
"Well, what the hell. It's no big deal for them to pack it up. If you don't want it tomorrow, I'll heave it in the garbage. But just in case it might appeal, they can put it in a container."

When it arrived, it was beautifully packaged with all of the selected varieties within a clear plastic container, extra chop sticks, dishes of dip mixture, and fancy napkins.

"There now, see? You can have a picnic tomorrow."
"It's getting on my nerves, Ma."
"What, Mike?"
"The way I can't eat. Everything gets stopped part way down."
"What causes this, Michael? Does the doctor know?"
"Yes. Nothing can be done. Part of the parade."

We were quiet in the cab on the way home, despite the dreadful driving. We seemed to be rapidly speeding, swaying from one side of the road to the other, darting in among other cars, and rattling over TTC streetcar tracks until we thought our teeth would fall out. The driver kept watching us in the rear view mirror, and I'm certain that I returned a look that threatened murder and mayhem. I was too distracted to write down the driver's license number, but clung onto Mike's hand to keep him from falling onto the floor. Michael wondered aloud if this driver was attempting to kill us, en route.

"How did you take that trip, Ma?"
"Not good. And you?"
"My back and tail bone really ache. This tired tummy is sure turning. Think that I'll have a hot bubble bath and soak in it. Once I get settled, could I have some hot milk?"
"My pleasure!"

Michael prepared his hot bath. I brought him a mug of hot milk, and then he asked,

"Mom, can you bring your prayer candle in? Place it on the toilet tank, please."
"Sure, dear. And do you want the light turned off?"
"Please, Mom. And can you put on one of my tapes for me?"
"You bet. Which one, Michael?"
"How about the Peggy Lee FEVER tape? The second side, with IS THAT ALL THERE IS? It'll automatically play the other side afterwards. Could you find the K.D. LANG tape, too? It's called ABSOLUTE TORCH AND TWANG. Put on side one, later, Ma. I like the first three songs best."

Michael had an impressive collection of records, tapes and a limited number of CD's. Much of the music was unknown to me. His taste ranged from heavy metal to classical, with everything in between. He had always been curious about music and wanted to know everything possible about the amazing variety available. His linguistic skills were also obvious in his collection. I couldn't even pronounce half of his albums. I found the first cassette, and Peggy Lee's HALLELUJAH, I LOVE HIM SO filled the dining room. Her warm, sultry voiced drifted into the bathroom, where Michael immersed himself among the bubbles. His inability to eat supper that night had depressed us both. It was, however, the first of many such meals.

NOT A TOTAL WASTE

Because I had missed spending Christmas with Michael, David and Kim decided that we would share a special dinner at Il Monello's, on Yonge Street that Saturday evening. Michael loved the filling starters and main fish courses offered there, so David humoured his taste buds. I had brought everyone small tokens which we unwrapped beside the fireplace at David's home, before leaving for the restaurant. He had opened a dry white wine from France for me, while they sipped their favourite martinis. Upon arrival at the restaurant, they surprised me with lavishly-wrapped gifts. I was thrilled with the hand cream and perfume from Michael and Kim. A large box, elaborately-wrapped with metallic paper and enormous ribbons, contained an ostrich-feather boa. David must have had a lot of fun selecting this unique, wonderful surprise. I burst into giggles and Michael sat there grinning. David and Kim looked mischievous.

That long, white, serpent-like coil of white feathers with red tipping had to be worn around my neck while we ate supper. The lewd effect was instantly hilarious. The entire restaurant watched this bizarre extravagance. Michael grinned and questioned me about my ability to eat my dinner while blowing away feathers. We shared an evening of zany humour. Since we'd missed out on the first festival season, we decided that we were celebrating the Russian Christmas. It cheered us to see Michael immersed in this nonsense and laughter. He ate very little, but he smiled frequently. For a short time interval, the tightness evaporated from his weary, wizened features.

CHAPTER EIGHT

Some free time was available to me during January when the students wrote their final examinations. I obtained permission to have a four day week-end with Michael, since I also had to visit a chiropractor as a result of a previous back injury. My arrival was a complete surprise. Although he had no fever at that time, his extreme exhaustion worried me. When I got to his apartment he was sleeping deeply, at seven in the evening. This was not unusual, anymore. However, the television was not turned on, and the apartment was in darkness. I tiptoed down the hall to see if Michael had gone out, or was sleeping. He seemed to be unconscious. He did not stir when I turned on the hall light. At first, it was difficult to ascertain whether or not Michael was breathing underneath his jade-green duvet. I shut the bedroom door softly, and placed my luggage in the front room.

I entered the kitchen and turned on the light. Cockroaches skittered everywhere. Dirty dishes were stacked on the floor, on the counter, and piled inside the sink. Garbage was loosely-tied in bags that spilled over onto the floor. The mess didn't deter me from just walking in and beginning the cleanup campaign. What frightened me was the realization that Michael had been too sick to handle any of this, obviously for over a week. It also meant that none of his friends had visited, because they would never have left this filth behind. I assumed that he had refused to answer telephone calls

NOT A TOTAL WASTE

except for mine, and had ignored the door buzzer. He had followed this routine previously, when he was terribly ill.

My mind mulled over the time when Michael had first told me of his positive testing for the HIV virus, and the soft smile which had played across his features as he explained that it was not necessarily a death sentence. We had agreed that "maybe it will never turn into full blown AIDS" or "maybe Mike will be the first one that doesn't die because of a medical science miracle." Reality hit me hard, as I looked over the mess which surrounded me in his kitchen. Now, time seemed to be fleeing our grasp. Mike deserved a legacy of respect and love which would provide him with control over the process of his personal dying. He must determine his care and treatment throughout this last passage of life. I must cope with his wish to remain in his own room, in his own bed.

Once the kitchen was in order, I went back to his bedroom. I stood at the doorway, wondering if I should disturb him. Michael rolled over in the bed, and faced the door.

"Sorry for the mess, Mom. What day is it?"
"It's Thursday, dear. I came to surprise you. I have the weekend to share. How are you, Michael?"
"Not good. It's just the usual explosive diarrhea and forceful vomiting. My chest hurts, Mom. The cough is worse. Swallowing is harder, too."
"Michael, have you talked with your doctor?"
"Nothing helps, Mom."
"Well, Mike, by the look of the kitchen, you sure have tried to eat. What would you like, now?"
"Baked beans with brown sugar. Milk. That's it."
"Coming right up. Anything else that I can do?"
"No, Mom. Except, maybe turn on the TV. Glad you're here, Ma."

He sounded wistful. I hurried with his food, and sat beside him on the bed as he nibbled. He suggested that we might want to watch the video ROBOCOP II to compare with the original. I went down the street to pick up a few groceries, and rented the film. We were both disappointed with the video, because nothing could compare with the director's style in ROBOCOP.

In the morning, I found Michael leaning against the kitchen counter around seven o'clock. He was mixing his DDI, and had already taken a shower. His effort to rebound was not easy.

"Is there anything special that you might like to do today, Michael?"

"Yes, Mom. I missed my Pentamadine appointment at the Rosedale Clinic. Could you call and make another one for me? Anytime after two o'clock would be okay. I'd like you to see if my dentist can check my gums afterwards."

"I'll call them shortly after nine o'clock, dear. The laundromat is open now, so I'll get it done while you're resting. Could you eat breakfast?"

"No, Mom. I just want to get back to bed."

"Not even a milkshake?"

"Okay, Mom. I'll try that."

He moved laboriously back to bed. He had no fever, but appeared wan and weak. He drank his liquid breakfast, and slept.

I sorted laundry for five machines, and sat reading the Toronto Sun and drinking coffee. I was alone in the laundromat at that early hour, but since it was Friday it would fill up rapidly. About twenty minutes later, four young men entered carrying large green garbage bags. I ignored them, until it was necessary to transfer my laundry to the dryers.

They had spread gold jewellery on the sorting counter next to the driers. Bracelets, chains, pendants and rings covered the length of the narrow counter. They were arguing over possession of a beautiful charm bracelet. I ignored their contraband sorting, and concentrated on the dryers. I knew enough about Metro life to keep quiet and mind my own business. Once I had all of the laundry moved into the dryers, I returned to the other side of the room, and sat down to continue reading my Toronto Sun.

Three more youths walked in with more garbage bags. I observed them as they dumped their bags onto the floor and started to sort jackets, shirts, jeans, underwear, socks--all new, good quality merchandise. It dawned on me that the police would be looking for these guys today. They seemed to have broken into clothing and jewellery stores recently. Nonchalantly, I continued

NOT A TOTAL WASTE

reading. I was alone. I knew that I was in danger. I also knew that I couldn't leave behind four dryers of Michael's clothing and bedding. By now, there were six young men, aged from sixteen to around twenty-five, sitting around the washers. They boisterously fought over their loot.

When the dryers began to run down, I continued to feed them quarters. I looked sideways towards the group. They stood brazenly staring back at me, stark naked. They had stowed every last vestige of their clothing inside the washers. They would be clean! I thought how much Toronto had changed over the years-- and those transitions involved more than the architecture.

Within the next twenty minutes I had completed my laundry. I folded clothes and newspaper and departed. These young men could have followed me, to ensure that I did not call the police. Concerns for Michael's safety were uppermost in my mind. He would never have been able to defend himself against a violent group like that one. I didn't speak of those naked Torontonian thugs to anyone, except Michael. He shook his head and laughed at me while I discussed the size of their biceps.

Michael's appointment for his Pentamadine treatment was set for two o'clock. We were on time. It took Michael about half an hour to complete his breathing of the medication, and I waited in the lobby. Sitting there, watching all of those beautiful, sick young men sign in, was depressing. Hearing them cough and retch over the treatment, was discouraging. Helping Michael stumble out afterwards, was disheartening. However, this drug worked to prevent pneumonia for many afflicted with AIDS, and that was truly a positive aspect. The humour and kindly compassion of the attendants at the Rosedale Clinic deserved commendation. How I admired them.

Michael's gum infections required some treatment. The thrush had also begun to develop, so we renewed his previous prescription. He was ready for a nap, by the time we got home. When he woke around seven that night, we made arrangements to go for a fish dinner. He couldn't complete his meal, but he did make a valiant effort.

We watched the video DIE HARD that night, and Michael teased me as I excitedly battered his teddy bear during the fast-paced film. After hot milk, he slept fitfully. His every movement woke me, as I heard the night noises echo down the hall.

In the morning, Anna and Jenni came over to visit and shop. I decided to drop off Michael's rust-coloured silk bomber jacket to be dry-cleaned, on our way. In his pocket I discovered some prescriptions which he had been given a couple of weeks previously. I told him that I would pick up his medicine when I was shopping. He seemed really pleased about that, and thanked me.

I went to three hospitals and four pharmacies, and none of them would release his medication to me. Finally, I went to a fourth hospital. They also explained that they could not locate Dr. Drake on a week-end, in order to verify the prescriptions. Since the pharmacy was actually closed to the public on week-ends, they could not provide me with his required medications. I stated that I was his mother, from out of town, and that he had been too ill to get these refilled earlier. When the hospital pharmacist stood her ground, I burst into tears. I asked her what would happen to him without the drugs. She replied that he must have them, or die. I asked her for the telephone so that I could contact the police to beg for help. I don't know what she thought of my reaction, but finally she said,

"Exactly how do you expect to pay for these drugs?"
"Plastic money, I guess. Do you want a cheque, instead? I have identification."
"No. Mastercard or Visa."

When I found that the drugs were close to $1000 I was in a state of shock. These were only a portion of the medications which Michael must have each month. Without them, he would die. With them, he would die more slowly. Hopefully, with less pain.

We returned home with his drugs as soon as possible. When I asked Michael why he had not picked up his medication earlier, he explained that he had lost his credit card and was waiting for the bank to replace it. I learned after his death that his card was lost when he had purchased my birthday gift. I felt a lot of guilt because of his declining health. I often wondered if purchasing my birthday gift had shortened his life span.

NOT A TOTAL WASTE

The day after Valentine's Day, three weeks later, I was able to spend four more days with Michael. His weight was now down to 120 lbs. and he was having serious difficulty sleeping. He had obtained some light sedatives from his doctor. He really needed something much stronger. We then discussed types of exercises which might tire him and make him sleep. His eating habits had not improved.

During the March school break, we shared four additional days together. The highlight was the purchase of a beautiful pair of black oxfords with large silver buckles on the sides. The paralysis in his right hand eliminated the purchase of laced shoes. We travelled to four different stores by taxi, trying to locate those special shoes. He was as proud of them as Sean had been with his first pair of Air Jordans.

Once he had purchased his new shoes, he decided that we ought to take a forty dollar taxi trip to North York. He wanted to shop at a prefabricated Swedish furniture factory. Their showroom displayed various items of attractive home furnishings. These could be purchased "knocked down" by the box and assembled at home. A modernistic, black-cubic television stand, containing three shelves and two oak-trimmed drawers, appealed to Michael. Once the taxi driver had lugged it down the stairs, grumbling under his breath all the way, Michael felt inspired. We would compile the pieces together to build his masterpiece.

That onerous experience reminded me of putting together numerous Christmas toys for Anna and Michael, many years before. Then, as now, we lacked parts, and directions were vague. Michael depended upon the French and German directions, since the English were too confusing. The assemblage was a four-hour exhaustive accomplishment. With pride, we installed the television set, VCR recorder, air filter machine, and a limited number of VCR tapes in the appropriate sections.

"Okay, Ma. Turn it on. Turn it all on. Let's see if the equipment will function on this remarkable podium."
"Podium? So this wobbly stand is now centre-stage? Oh, my God. Is the world ready for this?"
"Well, we can't exactly draw open velvet drapes to view our masterpiece, but we can turn on the power. With luck, maybe everything will function."

"Looks like it will. But Michael, what about your heater? It doesn't seem to be working properly now."

We had purchased a small space-heater that had a safety mechanism installed. This would automatically shut off the element, if anything obstructed the air flow. In order to re-activate the heater, it was necessary to insert a screw driver through a tiny perforation at the back. Neither of us noticed these requirements, and when the heater did not function, Michael was very discouraged.

"So now I have my entertainment hook-up, and no more heat. What next?"
"Let me look at it, son. There must be some small adjustment that could be done by an electrician."
"Forget it, Ma. Everything seems to go wrong at once."
"Michael, it's a good heater. I'm sure that we can find out what went screwy on it. I'll take it to the hardware store and they can fix the problem."
"Let it go, Ma. THERE IS NO NEED."

There was no reasoning with him, once he had used that expression. I vowed that I'd check out the heater later, when he was having a shower. Unfortunately, that didn't get accomplished. It was one of the many things which I tortured myself about later, with "If only I had..." expletives. The complete exhaustion which I was experiencing seemed to leave me numbed. Knowing how ill Michael was, I could feel myself almost withdrawing sometimes, in a desperate bid to control my emotions. It was as if I knew he was dying in front of my eyes, and I was afraid I would snap and start shouting disgusting obsecenities. As a result, I became quiet and more introspective than usual. Because Michael's circulation was not functioning well, he depended upon the additional heat of the machine each day and night. It didn't get fixed until my next trip down, and shortly afterwards it stopped working again. Perhaps the safety mechanism was too sensitive. Michael used flannel sheets and his duvet to keep warm, instead.

CHAPTER NINE

The next day, he had a trip scheduled to see Dr. Drake. He decided to go by bicycle, since the sun was warm and there was no hint of a wind. The weather didn't worry me. His weakened health state was a legitimate concern. He struggled gamely to drag the bike up the stairs and outside. I couldn't bear to watch him peddle away on his 18-gear, green "Mountain Bike". The only display of confidence which I offered was my restraint from hanging out of the front window to see whether or not he made it safely to the end of the block.

After doing "busy work" around the apartment, I sat on the couch near the front room window. On the pretense of reading, I could readily discern his approach from that vantage point. He returned within an hour, tugged away at the bike until he had it on the front porch, and unlocked the outside door of the apartment house. I knew nothing would deter him from dragging the bike inside, so I helpfully opened the inside door. I waited to welcome him at the base of the stairs.

"Hi, Mom. The doctor wasn't there. He has the flu, and his office was closed."
"I'm sorry, Michael. They ought to have called his patients to notify them. Then you wouldn't have biked all that way for nothing."

"You're right. I didn't realize how long it would take."

He started to manoeuvre the bike down the narrow stairs, when his leg became entangled with the pedal. Michael and the bike fell rapidly down the stairs. I reached to catch him at the bottom, and was slammed against the wall. Michael's right leg was torn from the knee to the ankle, and was bleeding profusely. Once the bike was installed against the front-room fireplace and Michael was in his bedroom, he sent me away. We were both in shock. Michael stripped off his jeans to determine the extent of his injury, and then called to me.

"Mom, can you give me a hand now, please?"
"Yes, Mike. How bad is it?"
"I'll need some wet and dry paper towels to clean away the blood. Can you bring rubber gloves? And antibiotic cream? Do you know where the bandages are kept in the bathroom?"
"Aye, Aye. I'll fetch them, master."
"Then be quick 'bout it, or it'll be twenty lashes against your stern...or something like that."

We both nervously laughed, and I rushed in with all of the first aid materials that I could locate. Michael had so little flesh, that the cut exposed the bone. Feeling giddy, I quickly pulled on the gloves and gently cleansed the area.

"Do you want me to take you to the hospital, Michael?"
"No, Mother. Just be very careful with the blood."
"I know, dear. But that's not a mere scratch. The blood seems to be everywhere. Don't you think it may need stitches?"
"No, Ma. Put the antibiotic cream on it, and stop making such a fuss. Can you bandage it?"
"Not artistically, but adequately."
"Shit. Just get the job done. Please?"
"Sorry, SIR."
"Mom, about the blood. I've been thinking, lately."
"Wow. That's different."
"No sarcasm. Just listen."
"Hmmm. I guess I'm just nervous about this leg, Mike. You know me--I sometimes react with silliness to try to alleviate the pain."

NOT A TOTAL WASTE 131

"Yours, or mine? Anyway, pay attention. What if the AIDS virus mutated? You know, any virus can alter or change its appearance. The results are similar in the disease pattern, but the virus shape is different. Can you imagine what repercussions that would have?"

I stared at him in alarm. "My God, Mike. The blood banks wouldn't be able to identify the virus. It could slip into the blood banks because they wouldn't be able to screen for it. AIDS would spread even faster. Even if they checked the blood of the dying, it wouldn't indicate the AIDS virus as they know it. That's a horrible concept."

"Sounds like a good monster movie plot. How to terrify the masses. An AIDS bug that they can't identify. But Mom, it IS feasible. If you were nervous about blood transfusions before, just consider those implications. What would you do to avoid contamination?"

"Damn. I guess if I have an accident, I have to take my chances. But, if I were having elective surgery then I could demand that my doctor draw some of my own blood ahead of time and save it."

"Good precaution, Mom. Stock your own blood at a blood bank. But what if some ninny mixed up that stock, by error? Mistakes can happen."

I felt chills up my back. "There has to be a solution, Mike. Aren't there hospitals that use cell savers? Don't those circulate the blood that's shed during surgery back into your body?"

"Right, Ma. Will you talk about those ideas to Dad and Anna? The AIDS virus could alter in strength, too. It could become genetically weaker or stronger. Nevertheless, it would still be a killer. If cold viruses can mutate, nothing could stop AIDS viruses from changing, too. Mom, I don't want you to die like this."

I looked closely into his eyes, blinked and looked away. His concern about the possible blood contamination was understandable, yet I could not respond to his final conclusion. He lay back on the bed and I managed to complete a tidy bandaging. I gave him juice and two analgesic capsules and he decided he would like a nap. I covered him up, because he was cold from the shock of the accident and left him to rest. I lay down for awhile, but continuously checked on his progress.

By seven that evening he called out,

"Mom? Aren't you getting ready to go out to supper? We're supposed to meet David and Kim at Brownes Bistro."
"Are you sure that you're up to that, after your space flight?"
"None of your lip, woman. Get ready for dinner. But if you have a few more pain killers and ice water, I'd really appreciate them."
"Coming up."
"Mom, I've been wondering. Would you like me to do a house design for you? I could, you know. I know the exact style of house that you would like. I have the time to do it now...and the training."

I stared at him. He lay in pain, recuperating in order to meet with David for an anticipated elegant dinner. Despite his discomfort from his leg injury, he pondered about a designed dream house for me. I looked into his eyes, and said softly,

"No, Mike. I don't want you spending your remaining time designing a house for me. I want you to use every moment to keep healthy and strong for as long as you can, instead."
"Are you sure, Ma? It would be a beautiful house design."
"I don't doubt that for one second, Michael. But let's be realistic. I'll never have the money to build it and that would make me bloody sad. No dear, not now. Use the time left for yourself and your friends. You could always write a book. You write better than any of those authors' novels stuffed into your shelves. Your offer of the house design means a great deal to me, Mike, and I'll never forget it."
"Okay, Mom. Love ya."
"I know, Mike. Thank you, son."

Michael hobbled through the evening, without a single complaint about his laceration. The leg lacked some degree of sensitivity due to the partial paralysis, but it must have hurt. Since I left the next day, I am not sure how much difficulty he experienced during the healing process. When I queried him about it on the telephone, he said that it was fine. Two weeks later, I observed that the leg was scarred, but healed.

On the day of my birthday in April, Michael sent a dozen long-stemmed red roses. They were a deep crimson, each bud perfectly formed. The vase was a green-tinged crystal. Tiny fragrant stephanotis blossoms were tucked in among the roses. I sat and held

NOT A TOTAL WASTE

one perfect rose in the palm of my hand, and wept. This would be the last birthday bouquet that Michael would send, and I was well aware of that. Memories of previous flowers, sent from diverse parts of his world, came to my mind. I took a Polaroid print of the flowers so that he would see how exquisite they looked on the coffee table. Bruce took one of me beside them, but my eyes were too puffed up and my nose red from crying. I was too vain to send him that copy. I telephoned him immediately.

"Son, the flowers just arrived. They're perfect. Thank you, dear."

"Now, don't cry. They're supposed to make you happy."

"They do, honey. Mothers always cry when they're this happy. You know that."

"Did they send you a good vase? I asked for that, because you don't have one."

"It's a clear crystal, with a tinge of emerald green."

"Oh, sorry about the green, Mom."

"Michael, it's lovely. It's your favourite shade of green, just as if you had selected it yourself. It looks as though it has always belonged on the coffee table."

"Okay. When are you coming down, Mom?"

"This Friday, dear. Right from school. I ought to get there by 6:30 or 7 again, if the traffic from Terminal III isn't too terrible. Is that all right?"

"Sure. It's just that...David and Kim arranged for your birthday party at Risha's. We worked on the menu--this will be very special."

"Oh, Michael. None of that was necessary. The flowers are enough. We could just take it easy and order in."

"Not for this party, Mom. I've been resting all week to be really up for it. We're all looking forward to this."

I assured him that I'd get to his place as quickly as possible Friday, and wear my best outfit. I knew that the evening would be incredible, and they did not disappoint me. The entire meal was amazing. I sipped a blood-red glass of Compari and soda, while the others chatted over their martinis and waited for the magic to begin. The first course consisted of a mound of finely-flaked chopped tuna, capers, spring onions, tomato sauce, a touch of dill and freshly ground pepper. It rested upon a bed of curled lettuce. The next course included steamed, miniature fresh-water clams, flavoured with a touch of garlic butter and parsley. Eight of these rested in their little shells around the edge of the plate, and at least a dozen were scattered upon a large serving of hot home-made spaghetti. Tiny chives and fresh oregano kissed the surface of this serving.

To cleanse the palate between the second and third course, a tall-stemmed dish of orange sherbert was served, with a fragile, rolled French pastry. Imported spring water was made available prior to the serving of a fine, dry white wine. The third course was baked duckling, sliced thinly into thumb-sized sections, with fresh, sauteed pears. These were arranged over a serving of cooked, fresh beet tops. Balancing the arrangement upon the plate was an attractively placed serving of fresh asparagus, miniature potatoes, petite artichokes, with a pear glaze. Each course was served with its own specific imported wine.

Even more exciting was the incredible birthday cake, carried on a large silver platter by the Chef. This was composed of numerous cream-puff shapes which had been filled with whipping cream and an orange-flavoured liqueur, called Grand Marnier. These were piled, one upon another, to form a large inverted cone-shape. The entire centre of this was then filled with whipping cream, laced with the Grand Marnier. Spun sugar was wrapped lightly around this confection, which sparkled as the light touched it. The taste was as impressive as the appearance. I had never seen such a triumphant birthday cake, and I crossed my fingers tightly as I blew out the single candle to make my wish. David had explained that the cake had been a very special order, which he and the chef had been planning for weeks. Phonetically, the dessert sounded similar to "crocquembouche". The Maitre D., the Chef and all of the waiters had joined our table in singing Happy Birthday to me, and then everyone shared in the pleasure of eating this gourmet delicacy. No-one else could have experienced such a birthday repast!

The rich cappuchino held an ounce of Frangelico liqueur, and I knew that I would sleep deeply that evening. David and Kim enjoyed a raw Italian spirit which sounded like 'grappa', and Michael had Earl Grey tea. Near the end of the meal, I noticed that Michael's rust coloured silk jacket was missing. Before I asked him about it, I realized that he had tucked it underneath the base of his spine for comfort. His face bravely showed no vestige of discomfort, and he had gallantly lasted for a four-hour episode of eating and

NOT A TOTAL WASTE

laughter. When I begged fatigue to get us both home, everyone jubilantly insisted that I open my surprise gifts, first.

David had purchased a miniature jade and brass box, which contained tiny moonstones and an uncut diamond. Kim had found an antique, intricately-carved Chinese opium bottle in pink coral. They both knew that I loved diamonds and OPIUM perfume! Michael's gift was saved for last. When I opened the red, heart-shaped velvet box and saw the antique Greek-style gold ring I could not speak. A central oval-shaped ruby was encircled with square-shaped rubies, which were surrounded by diamonds. Michael had selected this himself. David had helped him to go shopping, but as soon as Michael had seen this one, very special ring, he purchased it. I nearly fell off the chair. It overwhelmed me, and I was reduced to staring and gasping.

"Oh, Michael. It is so very beautiful. Wherever did you find it? It's just a dream ring."
"Glad that you like it, Ma. You deserve it."
"Oh, honey. It's just so beautiful."

Of course, I cried. I have worn it since, rubbed it with my finger when I am particularly forlorn and lonely, and watched it sparkle when the sunlight is reflected from the beautifully cut stones. Michael knew that my weakness has always been rubies and diamonds. Some women love other jewels; I have no idea why these two are my passion. It was a gift that cannot be matched, ever.

The ecstasy of that pleasant evening carried memories of sadness, as well. I did not ascertain until four months later that Michael had lost his credit card while puchasing that ring, and done without his medication for a week. Such a deprivation had not been any asset to his precarious health state. This knowledge added to the painful guilt often carried after the death of a loved one.

Wondering how I might have protected him more efficiently, or in some manner prevented the illness from invading every crevice of his body, or kept him alive a little longer, tortures me continuously. I wish that I had been able to take bolder steps to urge his rehabilitation. I blame myself because he didn't eat enough, often enough. The sorrow of watching a loved one's destruction from a terminal illness cannot be alleviated.

My trips were more frequent to be with Michael, now. Within two weeks I returned to spend May 3rd to May 6th with him. I had attempted to cajole him into taking a short trip to Barbados with me, while he was still strong enough. I thought that the warm sun, beauty of the ocean, flowers and fresh fish would entice him. He humoured me for a few weeks, and stacked up the clippings which I mailed. I suggested that instead of going with me, he might prefer to coax Ted to share the trip. I sent funds to take care of their expenses. He had tolerated my ideas until that first May week-end, when he said,

"Look Mom, forget it. I'm not going anywhere."
"Michael, you don't have to go to Barbados. It's just one of the places that I had in mind. The Causarina Beach Club, on the south coast is clean, and it has a decent-sized pool, too. You could rest a few days, and then take in the discos along the St. Lawrence Gap. The flying fish are tasty, and the water is safe to drink. It would be a change for you. You'd love having dinner at Pisces, or The Witch Doctor's. It would do you good. The sun would be warm on your body."
"No, Mother. Ted is going to Mexico for his holiday. I can't take the food nor the water there. Anyway, just let it go. I won't be travelling anymore. THERE IS NO NEED."
"I see. Michael, will you come home with me, for awhile?"
"No. That wouldn't be a good idea."
"Father agrees with me that a visit might rejuvinate you after the long winter. I could look after you better, up there. You wouldn't have to stay long, dear. I realize how claustrophobic you get in that small city. But, just a few weeks could help you to feel stronger."
"Don't think it's any use now, Mom."
"Michael, I could take you up on the plane with me this time, and bring you back in a few weeks, or whenever you need to see your doctor."
"Please, Mom. I'm fine here. My friends and medical arrangements are established. Leave it alone, Ma."
"Okay, dear."

I left the room quickly, because I didn't want him to see me cry. He was adamant. He would do no further travelling. He would not come home, ever again.

NOT A TOTAL WASTE

I went down to see Michael within ten days, because he had missed his doctor's appointment. When we conversed on the phone, he sounded disorientated and confused, which frightened me. I knew that he preferred to be in the disarray of his own apartment, no matter what. However, the decline in his health scared me, because he could not fully cope all alone. I approached him again about a nurse, home maker, companion, or entry to the Casey House Hospice. His temper was quick and unyielding.

"Look Mom, I don't want to go to Casey House. You promised me when I was in the hospital that I wouldn't have to go through that. There is no active treatment at the hospice, and I don't want to die at Casey House. I made it very clear to you that I wanted to be in my own apartment, and in my own bed. I don't need a nurse. Anna and you telephone, and my friends check on me daily."

"I just thought that your meals might be more nutritious, or that any other need could be handled more easily for you. They're very kind at Casey House, son. There are also volunteers who would help you. Your bowels are giving you so much trouble, again. Michael, this disease is messy, and you need any assistance that you can get. I hate for you to be alone at all, now."

"Ma, I have the phone beside my bed with the automatic panic button. I have Lynda and Ryan upstairs if I need to get help. David, Corey and Ted have keys to let themselves into the apartment, if they are worried. I neither need, nor want, a nurse. Do you understand?"

"What about a hired companion?"

"No. I'm not paranoid, but why bring in strangers, when I want my privacy? How do I know that I can trust them completely? I'm safer this way. Look, Mom. I cannot eat much food, anymore. I prepare what I need. I'm all right."

He lay back against the pillows, and coughed with a dry, hacking sound, and closed his eyes. The argument had left him spent and limp. I would defend his right to do things the way that he had requested. His demand for any small measure of control for his personal dignity, was evident. Michael deserved the right of free choice. Reaching that decision had not been easy, for either of us.

Michael was capable of facing the end of his life cycle with a rational attitude. His courage was not mine. My own feelings were unstable, particularly when I was alone. I felt vulnerable, and alienated. Studying the disease helped to provide a semblance of sanity. I crammed any book that I could find, trying to comprehend what symptoms to expect, what elements of AIDS that we were fighting, and why we were losing the battle.

CHAPTER TEN

Michael's long fight with parasitic toxoplasmosis dramatically affected his reasoning abilities, when linked with recalling chronological events. The doctors had assured us at the hospital that medication could reduce the toxoplasmo gondii effects. However, the disease would recur if the treatment was withdrawn. The long-term effects of the drugs could further undermine Michael's immune system. He could also suffer kidney damage.

One of the most potent viral infections that hammered at Michael's body was cytomegatovirus, which the doctors called CMV. It was one of the causes of Michael's failing eyesight, the inflammation of the esophagus, and the pernicious diarrhea. This infection was responsible, in part, for Michael's right-side paralysis. The neurological damage caused many changes in his body. This slow, painful, wasting death was common with CMV infections.

Because Michael's immune system was so badly weakened, opportunistic infections invaded his body. He was vulnerable to the Kaposi's sarcoma, a cancer cell which originates from the cells of the walls of the small blood vessels. Those purple-coloured cancerous lesions did not appear on the surface of Michael's skin. He was not disfigured, but his skin remained smooth and silky to the touch. However, they did invade his eyes, mouth and throat, lymph nodes and gastrointenstinal tract. Those life- threatening cancerous lesions became hard, raised surfaces in his throat and internal organs, so that he could not swallow. Those lesions were responsible for his constant choking when he tried to swallow food. Chemotherapy and radiation treatments additionally suppressed his immune system.

Multiple relapses caused Michael delirium and high fevers. Uncontrollable diarrhea destroyed his ability to absorb food nutrients, so that his weight dropped steadily. He was basically starving to death. Malnutrition and dehydration were combined with a dry cough, abdominal cramping and swollen lymph glands. His bed was frequently soaked, because of the nocturnal sweating. He suffered chills, fever and considerable pain. All of these problems only worsened, as time went on.

From May 16th to the 25th, I spent additional time with Michael. He had forgotten to see Dr. Baker at the hospital. When I arrived, I made another appointment to have his CAT scan, X-rays and blood testing completed. He also needed another Rosedale Clinic appointment for his Pentamadine appointment. He simply wasn't well enough to take care of these things alone, anymore.

"Mom, I'm losing track of dates, of what day or week it is. I get so tired sometimes that I can't remember if I've had something to eat or drink."

"Michael, this is the reason why I wanted you to have help here. I know that your friends and family call and remind you of your day-to-day responsibilities. But I still want someone with you on a regular basis, to take care of your needs as they come along."

"Look, Mother. THERE IS NO NEED. Will you please make certain that Corey gets all of my medication? I've stopped taking it. The doctors know of my decision, just in case you're in a panic about negligence. It's my choice, Ma."

"I see. I didn't realize...and you want Corey to have your pills, the AZT and your DDI? Maybe he'll come over, and you can give them to him yourself. It would mean more, that way, dear. He'll be more encouraged to take care of himself, for as long as he can."

I had trouble dealing with Mike's refusal to persist with his medication, yet I understood how overwhelming the disease effects were upon his body, mind and spirit. Mike would stubbornly make his own choices, and I hoped for sufficient strength to support him.

NOT A TOTAL WASTE

"You're right. I'll leave them on the dresser beside my bed for now. And Mom, you know how you always leave extra cash on my dresser? The money that you leave in case I can't get to the bank?"

"Yes, son. What about it?"

"Look, at the end, I want you to promise me that you won't count it--that you'll just put it in an envelope."

"Not count it? Put it in an envelope? Why?"

"For Corey, Mom. Not for right away. Save it for him for later, when money starts to get tight for him. He'll need it, Mom."

"Okay."

"And Mom, please keep in touch with him afterwards. You know, when I'm gone. He'll need you, too."

"If he'll let me, dear. I promise."

"And Ma, what about David?"

"I don't know what you mean. What about him?"

"Will you stay with David when you come back to Toronto?"

"No, Mike. I couldn't impose on him like that. He is a very private person."

"You could stay with David, you know. Because..."

"No, dear. I love David, too, but I just couldn't stay at his home. I can stay in a hotel, and if he has time, maybe I can meet him for lunch, tea, or supper--whatever."

"Okay. But, promise me, Mom, not to let that friendship drop. You can't withdraw and hide in your shell, once I'm not here. David is your friend, too."

"Not to worry. It's a promise."

"And Ted? And Corey?"

"Don't give it another thought. I'll keep in touch with them both--and Ryan and Lynda, too. Okay?"

"All right, Ma. Good."

He settled back onto his pillows, and absently stroked the fabric of his duvet. I watched him quietly and he seemed lost in his own thoughts.

The next morning we went to the hospital, where Dr. Baker has her office and clinic. Michael went through the CAT scan, a sputum test, blood tests and an X-ray series. We went to her office to complete his appointment. Four hours had been used up and Michael was exhausted. No wonder he had not arrived here last week. He was not strong enough to do this alone. Michael went into the office, while I sat in the waiting room.

Surrounding me were young men with AIDS, in various stages. One man, blinded and crippled, sat disconsolately in a wheel chair. Another leaned on metal sticks to keep mobile, and his face was badly discoloured with Kaposi's sarcoma lesions. He had no hair left because of the chemotherapy and radiation treatment. A third young man's body was severely wasted, perhaps from the cytomegalovirus, like Michael. He sat rigidly staring ahead. Another young man was dressed like a jogging enthusiast, and seemed to be so healthy that he appeared out of place. He had thick red hair, and his lime green shirt stretched tautly over his athletic body. He seemed restless at being in this room, and shifted about in his chair. Across from me sat a young man that reminded me of a younger, stronger Michael. I could not refrain from looking at him from time to time, nor could I stop my eyes from filling. When Michael returned to the room, these two looked closely at one another, recognizing some powerful similarity. Dr. Baker called me into her office next. She seemed very tired, and subdued. I wondered about the stress of her practice, and how she avoided complete burnout. Dealing with only AIDS-related illnesses must have been a tremendous strain emotionally, and physically. So few doctors had her courage and strength.

"It's good to see you, Doctor Baker."

"Thanks. Michael has told me that you're visiting him frequently."

"Yes, and the number of those trips has been recently escalating."

"Has he told you anything, about the level of his health?"

"He's explained his decision to cease all medication. I wondered if that was wise, since it is possible that he might have a bacterial infection in his bowel. It just seemed so premature for him to be giving up. The problems which he is experiencing now might be a relapse. Last time, the drugs which you prescribed helped him. Also, his nerves are frayed. He is using a light sedative and tranquilizer. His appetite is nil. I wish that I could coerce him into eating more. What are we talking, now?"

"Not long. Quality time, maybe a month maximum. He could manage up to eight months in hospital, using everything at our disposal. On the other hand, he could have a stroke, become completely paralyzed and bedridden. His vision is affected; he is becoming blind. You can expect a possibility of seizures, or even a coma. He is badly wasted now, and there is a definite possibility of dehydration. The vomiting and diarrhea will not disappear. There are growths in the bowel, throat, and abdomen. His lungs are filling up with fluid. We want him to have more checks on that, to verify that there is no tuberculosis. You should bring some feces in for examination, too."

"How is Michael responding to all of this?"

"Not the normal reaction. Most of them continue to fight. He has decided that he will not tolerate any more pain."

"What can I do?"

"Prepare yourself for his death. I'll send Paula to see you about counselling."

"No, that's not necessary. We'll be able to handle this ourselves, independently. Michael and I have already talked about the way he wants things to be at the end. He doesn't want counselling--you know how private he is. Thanks, anyway. For everything."

She called Michael into the office once more, and then gave him a list of appointments and prescriptions.

"Come on, Mom."

"Where do we go now? To check for TB or the feces analysis?"

"Neither. We're going home. Fast."

"Michael, if you have TB or a bacterial infection, maybe we could find treatment and get you stronger."

"You heard me, Mom. Come on."

I followed him out of the building, where a cab was discharging a passenger. He hailed that same cab, and we headed for home. The phone rang insistently, as we walked down the hall, once we returned home. It was the social worker from the hospital. Paula wanted to know if Michael and I would like to have counselling, either by ourselves or within a group. I thanked her, and said that we would be just fine, alone. Michael was too weakened to participate in anything like that, and I seriously felt that no-one could help me to feel any better. My world was falling apart, and I couldn't grasp a corner to hold on. How could I act calmly, as though nothing was bothering me? I felt as if a high, piercing 70 decibel noise was rushing through my head, and would suddenly be emitted through my ears, if not my mouth.

"Was that the social worker, Mom?"

"Yes, dear. I told her thanks, but no thanks."
"Good. We can face this death ourselves. A death with dignity, Ma. No machines to breath, eat, drink or defecate for me. Enough. THERE IS NO NEED." He lifted his chin defiantly and set his mouth in a firm grimace.

I sat beside him on his bed, hugging his white plush dog. How much I wanted to hug him, instead. He sat so rigidly, so proudly, propped up against his pillows. I hoped that I would not disappoint his faith in me. His privacy and independence were all that he owned. Please, God, please. Help me to have Michael's strength of purpose. He deserves to have some control over his situation. Help me to just hold on.

Early Saturday morning, after the usual laundry and tidying operations were finished, I opened Michael's door. He was propped up with pillows, and wide awake. Because of the worsening chronic cough, he rested more comfortably if he used a wedge-shaped form of pillows behind his upper chest.

"Hi, bright eyes. Would you like lunch?"
"I think I could try."
"The usual--baked beans, brown sugar and milk?"
"Yes, please. With a few thin slices of fresh English cucumber."
"Sounds exciting. Next thing, you'll want Oreo cookies. Then what would you like to do? Go shopping?"

I was teasing, of course. He resembled a weak, spindly kitten, but I had expected him to throw back some witty bit of sarcasm. David and Kim had invited us for supper that evening. That would be a major undertaking for him, considering his lack of stamina. He was brave to even consent to attend. His weight was 115 lbs now, and he walked like a sweet, shuffling old man. It was hard to accept that he must force his right leg forward, with a sort of kicking stride. The paralysis was worse in both right hand and leg. He had admitted that the tingling sensation had ceased. Now there was neither throbbing nor itching. There was just no feeling at all. His carriage had always indicated proud militance, but AIDS had stooped and aged him. He became riled when waiters mistook him for my husband, rather than my son. He would squint his eyes and glower at me.

NOT A TOTAL WASTE

"They're getting on my nerves, Ma. I might look haggard, but I sure as hell don't look as though I were the age of my own Father. It's a wonder that they don't tell me I've got Alzeheimer's."

"Hmmm. Did you read in the paper last night that some of the Alzeheimer patients over 60 years of age were found out to actually have AIDS-related illness? They were being treated for the wrong disease because of their dementia."

"You cheered me right up, Ma."

"Ouch. Didn't mean to say the wrong thing."

"Guess some folks are not appreciative of my fancy hair cut."

"I'm not commenting. You'll clobber me."

His light blond-brown hair had turned a dark orange-brown, which he hated. Chemotherapy and radiation had made it thin, as well, and it receded at the temples. He had tried every recommended technique, shampoo, cream, and diet to bring back his thick, wavy hair.

"Hard to believe that I modelled for a hair designer when I studied in Paris, isn't it, Ma? And did you know that Bob has pictures in his album of some amazing hair cuts that he designed for me?"

I remembered the photos of the sculptured, stylish hair cut stored within his photo album, but made no comment. None of the recent treatments which he had used could regrow his abundant tresses. He had defied society by using his electric razor and clippers. Michael had cut it to within a quarter-of-an inch in length.

"Yes, I remember those photos, Mike. I also recall the nude modelling jobs! Do you remember 'strutting your stuff' that summer in Vancouver at the nude beach with your friends? I heard all about that..."

"Oh, oh...my body was in great shape then, Ma. But what about this hair?"

"Well, it is pretty short now, Michael. Maybe if you let it grow a bit..."

"Mom, don't you know why I cut it myself? The only way that I can handle it is to use the clippers."

"It's just simpler, of course, and not as tiring."

"More than that, Mom. It's not that I'm lazy, nor am I trying to thumb my nose at society. God, Mom, I can't risk the fact that a hairdresser might nick my skin. What if I bled on him, and he had a small cut or scratch? He could get this damn disease from me. That's why I look like a hideous holocaust victim. Sorry, Ma."

"Oh, Michael. It didn't occur to me. I'm the one who is sorry. Besides, you don't look hideous. Just kind of stringy and spikey."

"Hmmph!"

Now, at my challenge to go shopping, he raised his head from the pillows, regarded me coldly and retorted,

"About that sarcastic crack regarding shopping. Yes. That's a good idea. You make lunch, and I'll get dressed. You can dial for the cab once I've eaten."

My bluff had backfired. I was stunned.

"Go shopping? Where?"

"I know exactly where I'm going, Mother. Hazelton Lanes. Get ready."

"Michael, it's expensive just to smell the air at the Lanes. What on earth do you need? Wouldn't someplace else do?"

"Is my lunch ready, yet? Shut my door, please, Mother. I intend to get dressed."

Sheepishly, I closed the door and prepared lunch. Serves me right, mentioning such a foolish idea. This gaunt, angry young man was definitely not physically strong enough to go shopping. His willpower, however, was a different matter. I marvelled at his conviction and control. What on earth would he purchase from Toronto's most expensive shopping district? I stopped composing mental arguments, and bowed to his wishes.

When the cab arrived, Michael gave specific directions to a selective men's wear shop. Once at our destination, I paid the cabbie, and assisted Michael to his feet. He defiantly pushed himself up the stairs by using the banister. I stayed behind him, in case he should stumble. I was trying not to get weepy, because I was frankly afraid that he would hurt himself. He should be in bed! I was so nervous that I felt giddy and slightly zany.

"Go in front of me, Mother."

"No way! I'm bringing up the rear. It's still cute, even if it has become smaller. Isn't less, more?"

"Woman, control yourself."

NOT A TOTAL WASTE 147

He gave me the expected scowl because of my tasteless remark. Then, Mike went directly to the sales person. He asked if he could try on one of the exquisite Italian silk shirts, displayed on mannequins in the front window.

"There is only one shirt that might fit you, of the three, sir. It's a size 15 1/2 neck. The others are 17 and 17 1/2."
"Which one? That one in the middle?"
"Yes. The others are too large."
"Hmmm. I liked the blue silk one on the left better, but let's go with the 15 1/2, then."
"I think I should tell you, sir, that the shirts are extremely expensive."

Michael gave him that dead-pan stare of his. He also managed to illustrate his famous scowl, albeit a little comically because he was so emaciated. In a low, contemptuous voice Mike replied, "I am cognizant of the price, thank you."

I walked away from them, then, and went to the opposite side of the elaborately-designed foyer. I gave the appearance of relaxing on the leather-padded divan. I reminded myself that this was not my business. I trusted Michael explicitly. He had made up his mind. Besides, I'd learned that once he had a predetermined plan, there would be no thwarting him. He was wearing his stubborn, "Let me do it by myself" look, which I saw first when he was four years old. This shirt was particularly important to him. When the shirt was brought to him for approval, he decided that he would try it on and disappeared into the fitting room for ten minutes. I worried about how he was getting dressed with a paralyzed hand, but since he dressed himself at home I stopped pondering. Michael had always been punctual. Whatever time he took to change, was obviously necessary.

I pretended to read a fashion magazine, while I mentally willed him to "please hurry". Nonchalantly, I checked the time, and judiciously watched the door to the dressing room. I was relieved when the mirrored door opened, and Michael reappeared. He wore the most splendid shirt I have ever seen, with his pair of baggy, worn jeans. He staggered a bit as he moved forward, stopped and grinned at me. I guess my mouth was hanging wide open. The colours were flamboyant and rich, in vibrant, glowing colours. The drawings on the silk shirt fabric, by the artist Gianni Versace, were boisterous and jubilant.

"Well, Mother, how do you like it?"
"Oh, Michael, it is the happiest shirt that I have ever seen you wear. My God, it is beautiful. The combination of red, gold, green, purple, black--it is a shirt of many colours. It's a rainbow shirt. What do the drawings signify? Michael, it is truly magnificent!"

Michael raised his left arm and indicated the many figure sketches on the sleeves, and front panels.

"These drawings represent the various acting performances which the artist has completed throughout his entire lifetime. He is a visual artist, fabric designer, fashion artisan and a Thespian artiste. There are only two shirts like this one in the world. The artist has one, and now I have the other one."
"How do you know this?"
"I saw Versace interviewed on a documentary the other night. Do you like it, Mother?"
"Michael, it is the wildest, 'most fun' birthday gift of all time. This is a real 'to-you-from-you' kind of extravagance, that you will have a lot of pleasure wearing. Go for it. You can wear it for your birthday dinner with David and Kim. It'll be perfect. Oh Mike, it's just gorgeous."

He grinned like a happy little boy, and that pinched, old-man face glowed with delight. He walked over to the clerk and handed him his Visa card, with a flourish. I imagined that the shirt must have cost a few hundred dollars. I had no real idea of the financial value of that one unique, portable art work. The following Tuesday he would be thirty-three, and he would wear this joyous new shirt for his birthday party. It would be his last hurrah--his defiant middle finger to fate. No-one deserved such an obviously gleeful shout, more than Michael. He wore it home in the taxi, sitting far away in the opposite corner, lost in his own thoughts.

CHAPTER ELEVEN

Once we were home, Michael removed the shirt and hung it lovingly on a padded hanger from his closet.

"Do you have a good silk blouse, Mom?"

"Yes, dear. I have that pure silk black one with the soft necktie and full sleeves that you gave me for my birthday about seven years ago. I take good care of it."

"Well, now you'll have another one. You're to wear this when I am dead, Ma. It is not to be my shroud. You can use it at Christmas, on your birthday--forever. It will fit you. Ma, I want you to use it. And I'll be there, with you, too."

I nodded, to show that I understood his wishes, but I remained silent. I struggled not to weep openly, as this was not the time, nor the place. This was a shimmering shirt of promise, and much love.

Michael walked towards me, and I stood still in the middle of the dining room, with my arms wide open to receive him. He hugged me gently, as if I were a fragile flower. I enveloped him and pulled him tenderly close, rubbing his back in a circular movement with the tips of my fingers. He chortled, and rubbed my back in the same way. We kissed cheeks, parted and smiled lovingly into each other's eyes.

"Unhand me, woman", he said, and I moved to let him stagger back towards his bed.

Michael drank a mug of hot milk and then slept until seven o'clock. He rose and prepared himself, without a reminder, to have dinner with David and Kim. He wore his beautiful brown-striped cotton shirt, a matching silk tie, and his rust-brown dress pants, with brown leather penny loafers. He looked rested and handsome. He no longer wore his contacts, because of eye tissue dryness, and a gradually restricted vision. He used his "John Lennon" tortoise-shell spectacles that suited him so well. As usual, he wore his Italian wrist watch which David had given to him when he had graduated with A PLUS marks from Teachers' College.

His rust silk windbreaker which he had bought on his last trip to Paris, finished off his outfit well. I was proud of the care he took with his appearance, and that his manners were that of a gentleman. I had located a creamy satin blouse to wear with my good black dress slacks, so I fitted in with the rich and famous.

The service, the food, the music, and of course the companionship, were superb. I couldn't have asked for a more enjoyable dinner with Michael, David and Kim at Risha's. It is an exciting place to dine. Sometimes we would notice theatre folk, political experts, vocal "artistes", business tycoons--people from the art world and financial sectors. We chatted, enjoyed the meal and the Mozart musical interlude, while I treasured this time with Michael. With concern, I realized that his face seemed extremely tense and tired. He had previously been in the bathroom for about twenty minutes. Upon his return, he had difficulty concentrating on, or responding to, our conversations. I leaned over and softly asked,

"Are you okay, Michael? You look a bit tired."
"No. The food wouldn't stay down, as usual."
"Look, dear, do you want to leave? Is it hurting you to sit this long?"
"Yes, but I don't want to offend David."
"He'll understand, son. He wouldn't want you in pain. Let's get you home. You've had one hell of a busy day. I've had all the food that I want. David and Kim can stay and enjoy the balance of the meal and relax. Michael, you just go ahead. I'll excuse us."

NOT A TOTAL WASTE

His face seemed to close up more tightly, his jawline became rigid, his eyes squinted, and then clouded with unshed tears. He did not utter a word, but looked steadily across the table at David and Kim. He seemed to be memorizing every detail of the evening, as if he would draw upon it later, alone. Then, he rose rapidly, turned and started towards the door. He moved so quickly that I was afraid he would fall. David and Kim looked up startled.

"I'm sorry--Michael's ill--I'll call--Thanks!"

I grabbed my coat and ran after him. I caught up with him at the corner of Avenue Road and Bloor, where he stood leaning against the utility pole, watching to hail a taxi. I put my arm through his, and said,

"It's okay, dear. They understand. They'll call you later on."

He turned his face away, and I raised my arm to signal the cab diver. We were home fairly quickly, and he went directly to the shower. When he was finished, I was reading the Toronto Star at the dining room table.

"I made some hot milk for you, dear. Feel like some?"
"Sure, but I'll get into bed first."

When I took Michael his mug of milk, he was propped up watching THE NATIONAL. He turned towards me, and looked at me steadily. Calmly he asked,

"Mom, what will you do with me after I'm dead?"
"I thought that you wanted me to cremate you."
"Yes. And then what will you do? Flush me down the toilet?"
"Michael! I will not."
"It's all right if you do, Mom. My career is wasted. My life has been wasted. My body is wasted. I guess I'm just a total waste. In more ways than one. Please don't have a funeral service here in Toronto. Promise me."
"Okay, nothing here. I had wondered about the Hart House chapel. You don't think it would be appropriate?"
"No, Mom. Nothing here."
"Is it okay with you if I have a service at home?"
"I guess it will be necessary, up there."

"Michael, your life has not been a total waste. You've been loved, and returned that love. Your own life has served as an example to others, in many positive ways. You've helped your loved ones to develop into better people. I'm not the only one who loves you."

"Uhuh. Right, Ma. I've had more than my share of rejection, too."

"I can understand that, dear. Everyone feels like a discard, once in awhile. Mike, you realize that Father will probably want you buried in the family plot, with all the rest of his clan."

"I don't care. You do what YOU want, Ma."

"Okay. Cremation. No church service here. But a memorial service at home. All set. Wanta boogie?"

"You are certifiable. You realize that."

"It's what makes me lovable."

"Sure, Ma."

I threw his plush puppy at him, grabbed his teddy bear for myself, and lay beside him on his bed. We watched a television documentary about the brutal political treatment of the Kurds. It horrified us both that after their involvement in the Gulf war, they were being abandoned by the country which they had aided. They were being literally murdered, a death through neglect, lack of food and cleanliness. The Kurds were educated, caring individuals, and their families were dying daily, one by one. It made us both angry.

"How can they be neglected like that, Michael? They're not getting assistance. Those families were used to a good lifestyle, and now they are treated like cattle."

"Well, Mom, the world doesn't offer much hope for its victims. Victims of war. Victims of crime. Victims of discrimination. Victims of killer diseases. You know--your minorities. Including the AIDS types. It's just another form of ugly racism, hatred, or whatever you want to call it. You know that it goes by different titles. Generally, society tends to grow deaf when they hear the cries of the dying. More than likely, there will be some responsible organization that will try to provide them with the tools that they need to survive."

"Not bloody likely. Not soon enough."

"Think I'll get some rest, Ma. Don't worry about the Kurds all night! You need some rest, too. Can you turn off the TV, please? And the light?"

NOT A TOTAL WASTE
153

A month after Michael's death, a receipt arrived from the Red Cross Society, and a beautiful letter thanked Michael for his generosity in sending $500 to use in assisting the Kurds. He wanted to do his part in rectifying that atrocity. He resented any active bigotry imposed upon citizens of his world. He had purchased acres of the Rainforest from the World Wildlife Society, and sent funds to support an adopted daughter in Senegal, North Africa. We now have accepted that responsibility for him, and struggle to translate her French letters when they arrive.

The next morning I did the laundry very early, in order to have some time with Michael before I caught the plane. At the laundromat, David surprised me by appearing with juice, pastries, coffee and the New York Times. We chatted for a little while about Michael's declining health, but I really had little to tell him. I was sure that he realized the reason why we had left so rapidly after dinner the previous night. Due to his sickness, Michael hadn't been able to eat much and his diarrhea gave him little rest. Perhaps my explanations were inadequate, but David was well aware of Michael's limitations. He left to take part in a squash game at his club. Depressed and exhausted, I finished the laundry and returned to Michael's apartment.

When I got back, I lay down for a short rest. Michael watched television and seemed relaxed. He had just finished lunch and we hoped that he might be lucky enough to keep it down. For some reason, I felt worn out and stressed. The tension was obvious in me, too. I rose and lit the prayer candle on top of the mantlepiece. Fervently, I beseeched for health and strength for both of us.

Just then I heard Michael stumble towards the bathroom, in a lurching, halting pattern. I knew at once that he had not made it to the toilet in time. The overwhelming stench swept down the hall. My poor Michael. I sat on the edge of the couch, waiting for him to make his way back to bed. It wasn't very long before I heard him call out in a nervous, high-pitched voice,

"Mom, I'm ba-a-a-ack!"
"Okay, honey. Just give me a minute."

I unclenched my jaws, and pressed my hands together tightly. Swiftly, I rubbed my hands together to warm them, and then placed my palms over my weary eyes to try to relax my eye muscles. I regulated my breathing carefully, and attempted to compose myself. The stress had been getting to me. I felt very defeated. No food seemed to remain in Mike's body. How could he survive much longer? The pain of dehydration and starvation must be horrible. He suffered constant cramps in his stomach, and in his limbs. His chest hurt every time that he breathed. He had refused morphine on his last visit to Dr. Drake, because he did not want to sacrifice the full use of his mental faculties. Michael demanded complete control over his decisions. This death would be done HIS WAY.

I walked towards his room, and I was utterly amazed. How could Michael possibly produce this much excretion, when he wasn't retaining any nourishment? The mess streamed from the bottom corner of his bed, and continued all the way through the dining room, into the bathroom.

"Oh, my God, Michael. Where is this all coming from? You have no food inside of you!"
"Sorry, Ma."
"It's no problem, son. I'm not really too great at this kind of clean up, but I'll give it a good try."

He said nothing, but just looked at me with wide, wild eyes. I wanted to bite my tongue off. How could I make a flippant crack like that? The copious amount of feces had flabbergasted me. How could his body create this amount? What was I really cleaning up? His weight was down to 105 now. Was this a portion of his actual insides? Was his body consuming itself? I wanted to scream and weep and kick the walls. There could be no catharsis for such an intense rage. I fought to regain some type of control. Then, I remembered that I had brought home a special deodorant powder from the hospital. Once it was sprinkled liberally over the floor, the smell was immediately obliterated. Slowly, I walked into Michael's room.

"Michael, I found this container of powder. Should you have any more accidents when I'm not here, dear, just dust it around. It takes away the smell and it is absorbed by the excretion. It's no big deal to clean up. I'll leave it on top of the toilet tank."
"Frankly, my dear, I don't give a shit."
"Pardon?"

NOT A TOTAL WASTE

"Sorry, Mom. It's from The Late Show. Hope I didn't hurt your feelings. It's a word play on that old movie. They just kept saying it last night. Frankly, my dear, I don't give a shit."

"Mike, I'm just unnerved by the amount of this stuff. You haven't been eating hardly anything, for so long. I don't understand where it all comes from."

"Just my guts breaking down, Ma. There's no antidote. I'm rotting inside, and it's coming out as garbage. Sort of like the computer line. You know, Mom. Garbage in, garbage out."

The tears stung my eyes, and I turned away. Maybe he was deteriorating to the point of putrefaction. God, help us. Please, help us. I pulled on the rubber gloves and tackled the final scrubbing in earnest. His bed required another change, so I asked him to step out of the bed for a few moments. He returned to the bathroom, and I got the bed completed. Michael returned, I tucked him into bed again, and explained,

"Michael, I'm going to dart over to the laundromat, and get these things done for you. The attendant will be there. She'll look after the washers and dryers for me. I want to go to the pharmacy down on Parliament to pick up some heavy-duty Gravol capsules. They'll ease the vomiting, and maybe they'll have something to help your bowels. Michael, I hate to go home and leave you this sick."

"Anna will be here in the morning. She takes the laundry home and returns it the next day, Mom. If I mess up again, she'll take care of it. Corey is coming over to-night, Ted tomorrow night, Tuesday is my birthday party with David, Wednesday maybe Lucy and Therese might come...I'll be all right. Thursday Anna is going to take me to see Dr. Drake, in the afternoon."

"Michael, I'm forced to be home for the next four days. The Department budget must be completed by Friday, the exams have to be verified and run off, and the semester marks have to be finalized. I'm sorry, Mike. I'm stuck. Can you hang on until I get back, on Friday?"

"Sure, Mom. Don't be upset."

"Would you like something to drink? Would you rather that I put some of the spring water in the refrigerator to keep it cold?"

"Frankly, my dear, I don't give a shit."

"There are a lot of juices in the refrigerator. Which one do you prefer?"

"Apricot juice. It's my very favourite."
"I didn't know that. On its way! And then I'll get going, to finish those few things, Michael."
"Mom? Frankly, my dear, I DO GIVE A SHIT."

I just backed out of the room, baffled. These comments were not at all like the Michael I knew and loved. It distressed me to hear him talk like this, but he didn't need me to retaliate. I found it best to walk away and disregard his festering fury. I did not know how else to respond. Anna would be in each morning, but I wondered how he'd get through the rest of each day. Despite the frequency of my phone calls and although his friends were taking turns to check on him, I worried that they might forget about him. He slept sixteen hours a day, and I knew that he could drift into a coma, experience a stroke, undergo a seizure, or go into a high fever. Any number of things could occur when he was alone. What if he fell, and broke a limb, or a hip? I wished that he would have permitted a full-time nurse, but he bitterly refused. When I hired anyone, he sent them away. I prayed that he would be able to cope, while I finished the essential tasks affiliated with my job at home.

I dumped the garbage bags full of laundry upside down into the wash machines, poured in soap, disinfectant, and stuffed coins into the slots. The surgical gloves and garbage bags were discarded into the waste receptacle. The attendant offered to take care of the laundry while I fled to the pharmacy. I gave her my change, and scooted towards Parliament Street.

When I explained the AIDS situation to the pharmacist, he kindly explained which over-the-counter drugs were the most potent available, without a prescription. Dr. Drake would return from his vacation on Monday, and I urged Michael to contact him.

"No problem, Mom."
"Michael, don't be so casual. You definitely cannot continue on this way. Would you let me take you to the hospital?"
"No. You promised that I wouldn't have to undergo all that experimentation crap again, Mom. I don't want to be a human testing device."
"They may be able to give you something to decrease the loss of body fluids, Mike. You probably need to have an IV hooked up. It scares me to see you in this state. You could dehydrate too quickly."

NOT A TOTAL WASTE

"Mom, not to worry. I have lots of help around me. I can also call Ryan and Lynda from upstairs if I need help. See? I just push this button for them, this one for Anna, this for you--and this one for 911."

"Michael, would you consider taking morphine to reduce the pain?"

"I can't take anything that is addictive, Mom. I'd lose control of my mental faculties. It would make me delirious and dependent."

"You have more guts than I do, dear."

"Not for long, Mother. They're all falling onto the floor, for you to shovel up."

"Damn it, Michael", I choked. "I just want to look after you properly. When you were a little boy, I could wrap you up in your quilted blanket and rock you to sleep in the big chair. You would relax, and nothing could hurt you anymore. I wish that I could just hold and rock you, until the pain was gone. I love you so much, Michael."

"Well, it's a damn good thing that there is no rocking chair here. I don't want to be touched right now. Not any more than is necessary. Every touch hurts, Ma. It's like the touch of death."

"Oh, shit. You mean when I touch you very gently, it feels like the touch of death?"

"Yes. When anyone touches me. I hurt too much, Mom. Everywhere. Please, don't cry. I love you too, Ma. I love you, too."

CHAPTER TWELVE

It was extremely stressful for me to leave Michael behind that first Sunday in June. He lay so still, with such a beatific smile, as I said my good-bye. I felt as though my soul had been sheared completely in half, for I was torn in two, leaving him behind. The responsibilities of my job must also be met. There was no alternative. Still, despite any job dedication, this was one time when I wished that I could tell them to stuff it. I wanted to be with Michael, instead.

On Monday night, when I arrived home from school, I placed my daily telephone call through to Michael.

"Hi Mike, how are you doing today?"
"Not good. Anna was here, and she took my laundry and tidied up the place."
"You sound distraught, son. Something wrong?"
"Mom, I just want you to know that on Friday, I am going to kill myself."
"On Friday? I'm coming to you that day, Michael."
"Yeh, well, I guess then you can do all of that stuff. You know. You can call 911 when you get here. The police, firemen and ambulance--you can just disrupt the entire bloody neighbourhood."
"Michael, please don't do this. What can I do?"

NOT A TOTAL WASTE

"Nothing, Ma. I want to apologize for using that silly expression from the Late Show. I didn't mean to hurt your feelings by saying, 'Frankly, my dear I don't give a shit.' It was meant to be funny, to make you laugh. You cleaned up so much shit."

"Oh, that wasn't important, Michael. Don't worry about that."

"It's important to me, Ma. And I also want to say that I'm sorry for anything that I've done to cause you pain."

"Michael, I love you so much. You have always been the best son that any Mother could ask for, and you've never tried to give anyone pain. Oh God--your sensitivity, your love--no-one else ever gave me the kind of support you do. You are the only one who understands me...what I am trying to do in education..with Father...with my life. You and I communicate in ideas, not words. You're such a big part of me. You're the best part of me. You're too hard on yourself, dear. You're so damned kind to everyone else, and ask for so little in return. Remember how traumatized you were when that mouse crawled into the toaster, and you inadvertently scorched him? Usually you caught the mice and let them go in the backyard. Hell, you wouldn't even let me use cockroach powder. Instead, I had to toss Bay Leaves all over the cupboards, to scare them away! I don't know anyone else who won't crush cockroaches. You've never hurt anyone on purpose. Oh, Michael, you deserve to live. To have a good long life."

"Mom, twice in my life I participated in unsafe sex. Neither of us used a condom. That makes me a potential murderer. I'm sorry, Mom. Please forgive me."

"Michael, did you know that you were HIV positive at the time?"

"No, Ma. I found out later. Both of them were tested and the results were negative. But what if they had been positive? Mom, I would have murdered them."

"Have your forgiven the person who gave you AIDS?"

"Now I have, Ma. It took me awhile. But I had to let the anger go. Whether I got this through the blood transfusions, or from someone during sex--they didn't know that they were giving it to me. It would never have been a purposeful thing."

"Yet you are judging yourself so harshly. Did you try to give those two people AIDS?"

"Mom, I told you--I didn't even know that I was carrying the virus. But it's a retrovirus. You know that it can hide in the blood and not be discerned right away. What if I gave it to them, and later on they develop the disease?"

"Stop punishing yourself, dear. Did you tie them to the bed and rape them?"

"Ma, of course not."

"Then, don't you think those two persons that you're so worried about were as responsible as you were, in a situation like that? They also practiced unsafe sex, by not using a condom. They were well aware of any potential consequences. And they tested negatively?"

"Yes, Mom. But that doesn't forgive the dangers and guilt, related to spontaneous sex. I cannot forgive myself. Will you please forgive me, Mom?"

"You were dealing with two consenting adults. They should have been educated enough to use condoms, too. Michael, there is nothing to forgive. Now, learn to forgive yourself."

"They were checked several times, later, Mom and they continued to test negative. No AIDS for them."

"Well, hopefully, they'll be practicing safe sex from now on. Look, Michael, people do party, drink too much, and forget. Spontaneous sex happens. It is a genuine hazard. It's a straight or gay worry. However, you did not set out to hurt anyone."

"I've never forgiven myself, just the same."

"God is not that judgmental, son. Forgive yourself, too."

"I'm just sorry for everything, Mom. I love you."

"You know that I love you too, Michael. Without limitations. So much."

"Mom, if you come early, please don't use all that resuscitation training you have. Promise me. LET ME GO."

"Michael, I promise. I won't call for an ambulance and take you to the hospital, either. I'll stick to your decision. There won't be any police, or coroner, or little red fire truck. I know that it is your wish to die in your own bed, in your own apartment. You have that right, son. But Michael, it won't be easy for me. You are my only, dear son."

"I can't take any more pain, Ma. I just can't. It has to end."

"I don't want you to kill yourself, all alone. Michael, I was there when you were born, and I want to be there with you, when you die."

"I've tried, Mom. I've tried so hard. I'm very, very tired."

"It's just that...I can't bear to have you die all alone. I want to be there, with you, to hold you with love. Michael, I want so much to help you go, gently into the night. Not all by yourself. It isn't right. It isn't right."

NOT A TOTAL WASTE

"I love you, Ma."

He hung up softly, and I sat in stunned silence. I did not know what to do, who to contact, or what to think. Then I trembled. I shook. I wept. Shortly afterwards, I called Anna and explained the phone call. She said that she'd call Michael right back, and would go over to see him, extra early in the morning. She knew that Ted, Corey and David were expected to see him during the week. I reminded her that she would have to take Michael to his medical appointment with Dr. Baker on Thursday afternoon. She said she would call me back, if there were any other complications.

I went slowly down the hall to the bedroom and lit the prayer candle on my desk. I prayed alone for about five minutes, and cried softly. I wanted to howl in pain, but it wouldn't have helped. Michael had reached the end of his life, and I had no safety net.

Death with dignity didn't necessarily include doing suicide, all alone and in great pain. What if he did something wrong, and made himself suffer more? What if he went into a coma and lay there unable to communicate? What if his brilliant mind was trapped in a paralyzed body for months or years? What if the drugs he took caused more damage and torture than he now experienced? It was illegal for me to help him to die. I could not even hold a glass to his lips, to speed him on his way. I was helpless to ease his burden of pain, in any manner. Yet, I could not think of him dying all alone--with no person nearby, that loved him. His physical pain was so great, that he could not even tolerate being lightly touched. He deserved to be cherished and held in loving arms, offered up to God with pride.

Bruce had been reading the sports section of the Toronto Star during all of this, and when I returned to the front room, he looked over the top of the newspaper and asked,

"What was all that about?"
"Michael said that he will kill himself on Friday."
He stared, and said nothing.
"I don't know what to do to make him feel more positive about himself. I don't know how to handle this."
"You've done all that you can. This is his decision, and it's out of your hands. The poor little bugger. Let him go."

"No. It can't end like this."
"He must be deeply depressed, and in a great deal of pain."
"I cannot believe that he will do anything rash. He will wait until his birthday, and until he has taken care of all of his good-bye's. That would include his appointment on Thursday with Dr. Drake. But I don't know what to think after that."
"Anna will see him tomorrow again. Check with her then. Maybe in the morning, he'll feel stronger."

I didn't know who to call, without imposing upon them. I remembered that Michael had not seen Lucy and Therese recently, so I telephoned Lucy. I reminded her that Michael's birthday was June 4th and asked if she could visit him. She promised to make arrangements with Michael for one evening during the week. However, she made it clear that she was provoked with me for neglecting Michael and leaving him alone. She did not comprehend that I had tasks which must be completed by due dates. Nor did she realize how much time I had been sharing with Michael. She said that I should have signed off sick and taken an indefinite leave.

The teaching profession is not arranged so that people just take time off whenever they wish, particularly since I had already been provided with a compassionate leave. She was disgusted with me when she hung up and I winced with guilt. There was no way to erase the torment which I was experiencing. I wanted to be with Michael for every last remaining moment.

When I called him on Tuesday, he seemed calm and loving. I kept the conversation as light as possible and Michael refrained from mentioning his suicide threat. He was looking forward to celebrating his birthday that evening with David and Kim. He would wear his amazing new shirt. I wished him a Happy Birthday. He said that he found the new electric toothbrush helpful and had noticed that his old plastic cutting board had been replaced with a marble one. He thanked me for his gifts and I wished him a great dinner.

When I reached him on Wednesday, his voice sounded strained and high-pitched with tension. He was upset because he had been too ill to participate fully in his Birthday Party the night before. Feverish and giddy, he had arrived late at Risha's--alone--by taxi. David had been dejected because the kitchen closed at ten o'clock.

NOT A TOTAL WASTE

Due to Michael's late arrival, the menu fare had been restricted. The well-arranged party had not been the anticipated success. Michael ate very little, was afraid that he might faint and create a scene, so he left within an hour. Michael had not explained to David the actual dimensions regarding his illness. He was too proud to appear to be complaining or whining. When asked how he felt, his response never varied from, "I'm fine." Michael's own frustration and rage about his disease, and his shame because he thought he had let David down, came through clearly when he said, "I messed up, Mom. I messed up my Birthday party. I JUST MESSED UP." I could hear his voice tinged with pain and tears. No solace could be offered.

I had immersed myself in my school work load upon my return home. It had taken twelve to fourteen hour days to be certain that I had covered every consequential detail. By Thursday afternoon, every task seemed to be completed. The administration and staff had given me plenty of support. Their empathy and compassion had been valued gifts. My students knew also that I was under terrible strain due to Michael's impending death and cooperated beautifully. I had not requested additional unwarranted time off. I finished the essential duties, and prepared for the Friday afternoon flight.

On the drive home from school on Thursday, I felt as though a dark cloud hung over me. My depression was intense and I drove so slowly that I was a highway hazard. Tears streamed down my face. I had lost control over my emotions. Once I arrived home, I tried to telephone Michael, but he did not answer. I remembered that he was going to see Dr. Drake with Anna, so I called her.

"Michael's not doing well, Mom. He kissed me outside of the apartment house and told me he loved me. You had better call him, Mom. Tell him that you love him, too, because..."
"I tried. He won't answer the phone."
"I don't know what to tell you, Mom. He's in a lot of pain."
"I'm going to call Dr. Drake."

I managed to catch Dr. Drake just before he left his office for the day. I detailed my concerns related to Michael, and he said,

"Michael was here. I honestly don't know how he made it. I had not expected to see him again, after his last visit. Michael has a lot of courage."

"My daughter Anna brought him."

"He is extremely ill. His weight is 100 lbs. now. You must realize that he has little time left."

"Yes, I know that."

"When do you intend to come back down?"

"Tomorrow, unless I can get a special flight tonight."

"I've seen that look...that I saw in Michael's eyes... before...in other young men, with this disease. Please get to him as quickly as you can."

"Thank you, Doctor. I will."

For some reason, I could not even tell Bruce about the call to the doctor, or why I seemed to move as slowly as a slug. He took me to dinner that night at the Holiday Inn. Because I knew that I had no appetite, I ordered eggs, toast and coffee. The solids stuck in my throat, so I just sipped the coffee.

"You must eat. You can't go on like this, without some food to keep up your strength."

"I would, if I could."

"What is wrong with you?"

"I can't explain it. I just have this terrible overwhelming feeling of foreboding. I sense such urgency, as if something is happening to Michael. RIGHT NOW. This very minute. But, I feel so ineffective. Something seems to keep me from responding, from acting. It's as though my body and mind are numb. What can I do to help him? ZIP! NOTHING. I feel so damned useless. I can hear his voice, calling me. Something is just very wrong, right now."

"Oh, it's that motherly instinct at work again."

"It's rarely incorrect."

Bruce nodded. Suddenly, I replaced my knife and fork onto my plate.

"Bruce, please help me. I feel as if I'm going to snap. To crack in half. Please, call the waitress over here. I want to start screaming. I have to leave. Please help me get to Michael. NOW. I'd run all the way if I could. I'm sick of being patient and nice, and trying to wait until Friday. I can hear him as plainly as if he were right here, beside me. Damn it, he's in trouble, and he needs me. CAN'T YOU HELP ME?"

"Don't panic. How can you get there? The last flight left at 6:10, and now it's 6:20."
"Well, there was an Air Canada strike during the past few days. Maybe another airline put on an extra flight to cover the overflow passengers. I could telephone to find out. I can't wait until tomorrow."
"Okay, if it will make you feel better. I just want it to be over. We'll go home, and you can check from there. If a flight is available, I'll take you to the airport."

I have no recollection of packing, or getting to the airport. I remember Bruce patting my shoulder and kissing my cheek goodbye. I sat on that tiny plane, nursing a rye and gingerale to settle my nerves and upset stomach. Tears flowed unchecked down my cheeks, and I blew my nose constantly. The stewardess avoided me and I didn't blame her. I had no desire to talk to anyone, but earnestly wished that I could make the flight move twice as fast.

When I indicated to the limousine driver that my son's life was in jeopardy, he took every risky short cut possible to get me to Michael speedily. My knees and hands trembled when I inserted the key into the lock of his apartment door. I was terrified that I had arrived too late.

"Michael? It's Mom. Mike, are you here?"

No one answered me.
I dropped my purse and overnight bag in the hall, and ran. No, Michael was not in his bed. No--not in the front room--not in the dining room. Why were all of the lights left on? Why was the television off? Had he just stepped out? I rushed to the kitchen, and found things in disarray. The bathroom was in utter confusion. Excrement covered the floor, toilet paper had been pulled from the roll and left in whirls about the floor. Michael's new white bathrobe was thrown in a dirty jumble. I couldn't see his old green one, his favourite, anywhere. The bath mat was pushed aside and formed a white, fluffy peak underneath the sink. A dark, dirty-coloured residue lined the sink. Michael's "John Lennon" spectacles lay abandoned on top of the toilet tank. Oh, please, God, help me. WHERE WAS MY MICHAEL? Where had they taken him? I checked the excrement, and it was still soft. Maybe he was nearby? Could he be upstairs with Lynda and Ryan? Maybe he was having

tea, and coming right back. Maybe he was already dead. MICHAEL, WHERE THE HELL ARE YOU?

The phone screamed shrilly. Startled, I ran and grabbed it.

"Hello? Michael?"
"Hi, Maria. It's Lucy. Therese and I have Michael at the hospital. We tried repeatedly to phone him, but he didn't answer. We left messages on his machine. If you play it back, you'll hear them. We finally came over."
"What do you mean? What are you telling me?"
"We knocked on the door and he didn't answer. So we went upstairs to Lynda and Ryan and got the key from them."
"Why is he in the hospital? Get to the point."
"When we found him, he was on the bathroom floor. We have him here, now."
"Will he be all right? Did you call his doctor?"
"We called 911 and brought him here by ambulance."
"You didn't call his doctor? All of the numbers are still on the kitchen cupboard door. Does that mean that the Police were here? The Fire Department? The Ambulance? Oh God, all that fuss and noise that I promised Michael would never happen..."
"Listen to me, Maria and listen carefully. He tried to kill himself. We brought his medication bottles here. He took seconal. Do you understand? He tried to kill himself."
"Why didn't you call Anna, or me?"
"He vomited up his medication. Check the sink, and you'll see. How could you leave him alone, for weeks at a time, like that? You know that he's dying. He must have been lying there for days. How could you neglect him? He didn't deserve to be treated like that. If we hadn't found him, he would have died, lying in his own shit."
"What are you saying?"
"If we hadn't found him, he would have died on his bathroom floor, from sheer neglect."
"No. HOLD IT. Just hold it there. Anna came for the last three days. I was here the previous ten days, straight. He has not been left alone. Check with Ted, Corey and David. Someone checked on him, each of the last three evenings. I even called you to ask you to arrange an evening to celebrate his birthday. It's the way Michael wanted it."

NOT A TOTAL WASTE

"He should never have been left. He would have died if we hadn't intervened. Wasn't his life more important than your career? Why weren't you there for him?"

"No. STOP THIS. Anna took him to his doctor this afternoon and brought him back about 4:30 or 5 o'clock. I don't know what happened then. I tried to get him at 5:30 and again at 6:20."

"Play back the telephone answering machine. You'll hear our attempts to reach him. We got alarmed. That's why we got a key and got in there."

"I talked to his doctor this afternoon. I got the next possible flight. Oh, God, not the hospital and 9ll...I promised Michael that I would never do this to him. Did you ask him if that is what he wanted?"

"He didn't say NO when we got him ready for the hospital. He wanted to live. We did what was right."

"In your mind. Not in Michael's. Bring him back here."

"We told him where we were taking him."

"Do you know how little time he has left to live? Did you know that he stopped his medication last week, and that he had notified his doctors of his decision? Bring him back here."

"We can't do that. The police are involved. This was an attempted suicide."

"That's the heartbreak of it. He has very little time left to live. Because you've contacted the police, he'll have to stay in hospital for psychiatric evaluation. I don't think that they'll allow him to sign himself out, or me to take him out, until he has undergone counselling. Up north--at home--they keep attempted suicides from three to six weeks in that ward. Oh, my God, he'll die there. In a psychiatric ward. Michael was terrified of senility, because of this disease. He was scared that the lesions would destroy his mental functioning. Dementia was his worst nightmare. Oh, please God, he didn't want to die in a psychiatric wing."

"You're not rational. I can't talk to you."

"Yes I am, damn it. I'm frightened. And I'm angry. You had no right to do this to him. He doesn't deserve to die alone, in a psychiatric ward. I promised Michael that he could die here, in his own bed, in his own apartment."

"We did what was right. We did what was legal. We'll talk to you some other time, when you make sense. You're totally hysterical. I don't have to listen to you, now. Michael's here, in the Emergency. We brought him here, because we care about him. We're leaving. I suggest that you get here."

She hung up.

I sluggishly moved my hand forward and put down the phone. Then, I heard a peculiar, high, keening sound. I could not comprehend its source. I hugged myself, wept and moaned. The sounds frightened me, as if they were coming from a great distance. I hugged myself tighter, tighter--trying to protect myself against that horrible noise that threatened to rip me apart. Then, I heard the phone ring again. When I cautiously picked it up, Bruce spoke.

"Maria, are you all right? Lucy called here and told me about Michael. She said you were hysterical."

"Oh, God, Bruce. She took Michael to the hospital. He tried to commit suicide with an overdose. The police are involved. They might never let me get him out of there."

"Can you get to the hospital? Can you go and see him right now?"

"I don't know. I can try. They'll put him in a psychiatric ward. He'll die there. Alone. He can't sign himself out. I think I'm going to throw up. Or faint. I'm so cold. I don't feel right. I can't do a damn thing to help him."

"Can you call me back? Will you let me know?"

"Let you know. Yes. Yes. I'll try. I'll call you. Pray, Bruce. Pray like hell. Poor Michael. Our poor baby. Please pray for him. Bye."

Why was I suddenly so angry at Bruce? Why couldn't he be here to help me? Why was I always left to take care of everything? Why was I wasting time whining? If I don't hurry, Michael might not be alive when I get there. Why wasn't I stronger? Why couldn't I be more effective, tougher, capable? How would I do this? Michael might live for awhile longer. How would I get him out of the hospital? HELP ME, GOD. PLEASE. HELP ME. I can't do this. I just can't.

SECTION 3

CHAPTER ONE

The phone rang again. I blew my nose, wiped my eyes and carefully, as if it were a deadly viper, I picked up the telephone.

"Yes?"

"Mom, it's me, Anna. Lucy called me. Will you be okay?"

"Anna, Anna. It's a bloody mess. Michael will never be able to get out of that hospital. Lucy put him in there. The police were there. He tried to kill himself. He'll die in a psychiatric ward. I don't know what to do."

"Mother, STOP. Lucy said that you were not rational. Stop. Pull yourself together. He's still ALIVE. Michael is depending upon you. Be calm. Get back your control. If you can't sign him out, then you'll have to play the doctor game again, Mother. One way or another, you have to get him out. Call a cab and get to the Emergency now, before they have admitted him."

"I think I've gone completely mad, Anna. I don't feel right. I probably am incoherent. Lucy is likely right. Anna, why didn't Lucy call Michael's doctor instead of making all of her own decisions?"

"Mother, calm down. Michael is Lucy's friend, too. She loves him, Mom. And he's always loved her. She did what she thought was right. Think about it. Penny, Lucy, Therese--they're hurting, too. Now, brush your hair, put on your lipstick and get to the damned hospital. You're the only one who can get him out. Call me back, after you've checked there."

"Yes. I'll try."

NOT A TOTAL WASTE

I hung up and stared at the phone. Suddenly, I refused to answer it again. Everyone dumped their expectations on me--what else was new? Oh hell, somehow, I'd get to the hospital. I'd play the doctor game. I'd use my Ph.D. and pretend it was an M.D. If I said that I was a doctor, they might listen to me. The only value in the Ph.D. degree, otherwise, was to get a taxi faster, or to get any available plane flight. Was I merely a distraught, hysterical mother? Was the promise that I had made to Michael the best route for him? Should I allow them to admit him to the hospital? They could care for his needs more appropriately, provide medication, and he could have an IV hooked up. The only certain solution required that I honour Mike's request.

I closed the apartment door firmly behind me and began my sojourn to Michael. I was half-way down the front walkway when I realized that my legs wouldn't propel me forward. I was mentally willing them to move me, but I remained petrified in one spot, holding onto the fence post. I felt dizzy and sick to my stomach. Where was this vertigo and nausea coming from? Ryan came down the stairs and reached me.

"Are you okay?"
"No. Michael is in the hospital. He's dying, Ryan."
"Dying?"
"The doctor told me this afternoon that he has little time left. He tried to take seconal to-night, and puked up black vomit. He must have been stockpiling all of his sedatives for awhile. He's alive, but how the hell am I going to get him out of the hospital."
"Why would you want to bring him back home? He's too sick, isn't he?"
"Ryan, I have to keep my promise to him. He wanted to die here, in his own bed. Not in a hospital. How can I help him, Ryan?"

He reached out and wrapped his arms about me, held me, and rocked me gently as I wept. He and Lynda were Michael's friends. They had all studied together at university, in Florence and in Rome. They had toured Europe and checked out artifacts and architecture there. They knew each other well. They would miss my Michael, too.

"Come on. You've got to get a grip on yourself. For Michael. I'll take you down to the corner and hail you a cab. You'll be okay once you get to the hospital. You're strong. Michael was always so proud of you. You can do it."

"Oh God, help. If only I could get him home."
"Do you want me to come with you?"
"No. Ryan, please help me to get a cab. I'll play my doctor game."
"What does that mean?"
"When Anna was in the hospital with a crushed leg, they wouldn't tell me anything. They wouldn't let me see her. I walked up to the doctors and introduced myself, using my Ph.D. degree as if it were an M.D. degree, and asked to see her X-rays. They showed me broken bones that were feathered and dog-toothed. Those pictures were horrible. I played the game and told them which bone specialist to call. I told them that the leg could not be pinned, nor any metal plates used. They could not understand how to stabilize the bone, either. Then I demanded to see Anna. It worked--until the bone specialist asked me who the hell I really was. I told him that I was just Anna's Doctor Mom, a Ph.D. doctor. At least I knew then, first hand, how severely smashed her leg had been. My acting got me past the nurses, and alongside of Anna. I was able to demand blankets for her, since she was going into shock."

Ryan tilted his head to one side and laughed.
"See? You've got your old spunk back again. You can do it. Now, go and get Michael. Bring him back home, as he wanted. Come on, here's a taxi for you."

By the time I got to the hospital I had stopped trembling, but I felt ice cold. It seemed that someone else had taken over my body, and was manipulating it. I felt distanced from everything. I held my head high, took a deep breath, and walked, robot-like, directly up to the Emergency counter. I hoped that I wouldn't trip and land flat on my face.

"I'm Dr. Smith. I understand that a young man called Michael was admitted by ambulance about an hour ago, with an overdose."
"Oh yes, Doctor, he's in cubicle four. Dr. Lee is with him."
"Fine. Thanks. I'll find it."

I walked to the draped-off cubicle, stood beside the open drapery for a few seconds, and tried to compose myself. The

NOT A TOTAL WASTE

panorama before me seemed unreal. The doctor was checking Michael's blood pressure. Michael's eyes were open, but his head was down. He looked desolate and completely forlorn. He was trembling violently as though an icy wind blew. I was concerned that he was starting an epileptic seizure. He looked up, saw me, and his eyes grew wide. A look of bafflement, and then a small smile, played across his features. I raised my hand towards him, motioning him to secretly remain silent. PLEASE MICHAEL, DON'T GIVE ME AWAY! I walked up to Michael and placed my left hand on his arm, to let him know that I was truly beside him. We both needed a touch of reality.

"Dr. Lee? I'm Dr. Smith. I'm Michael's family physician. I'd like to take Michael home now. Would you please instigate the completion of the necessary paperwork?"

"He has ingested seconal, Doctor. This was an overdose."

"Yes, I am aware of that. He did regurgitate them. No matter. I'll take full responsibility for him now. I'll take him home with me. I do not want my patient admitted. Would you get me a nurse, please?"

A nurse popped in, without being called. Dr. Lee watched me carefully, evaluating me cautiously through narrowed eyes. I smiled with false confidence.

"Oh, nurse, would you get me a wheel chair, please? I'm Dr. Smith, and I'm taking this patient home. Could you also telephone a taxi, if there's not one waiting outside the door?"

"Yes, doctor."

I had sounded so officious and poised, that I was impressed with my own performance. Was this the result of all of those female-assertiveness courses? Was this the time to play "lady bitch"? It was a matter of necessity that this charade work. I must get Michael out of this cubicle and back home!

"I'll take care of the paperwork, then, Dr....."

"Thank you, Dr. Lee."

When he left, the nurse returned with a wheel chair.

"Nurse, what is your name? You're not wearing a name tag. Why would you bring me a chair without foot rests, when this patient is partially paralyzed? He'll drag his feet and break an ankle from here to the door. Please fetch me a proper wheel chair, immediately. And is the cab available?"

She stared at me, turned and ran. Within seconds, she had the correct chair. She then helped me to ease Michael into his bathrobe and the chair.

"The taxi is waiting at the door, Doctor."
"Thank you for your help."
"Mom? Money. Costs about $35.00. Mom?"
"No problem, dear. No money problems, Michael. If only that would solve everything, darling."
The nurse's eyes studied me. "Mom?"
"Yes. He is my only son."
"Oh." Her eyes were suddenly filled with compassion. She understood. She patted my arm, leaned over to Michael and said,
"Take care, Michael. 'Bye."

As I pushed and pulled Michael in my efforts to get him into the taxi, two ambulance drivers opened the back of their vehicle, turned and saw Michael. They both walked over and said,

"Hey, Michael. How are you feeling now? Better?"

Michael recognized them as the attendants who had ferried him to the hospital, and replied,

"Oh, yes. Better. Now."

Once we were finally settled into the taxi and were started on our way home, Michael turned to face me. He grinned mischievously, waggled his finger at me, and said,

"Mom! Tsk, Tsk! Mom!"

I smiled right back at him, and kissed his cheek. I held his hand in mine all the way home, and prayed that I would have enough strength to help him. The next difficult problem was trying to move him down the stairs and into the apartment. He had no strength at all and was a dead weight for me. Despite his frailty, I could not carry him. I had to get on the step below him, lift and pull him towards me by grabbing onto the front of his old green bathrobe. I would shift him in this manner, lift and convey him down, one step at a time. Then, he leaned against me until I had transferred him to his bed.

NOT A TOTAL WASTE

Somehow, I removed his terrycloth housecoat. It was easier to just leave the blue hospital gown on him. I guided him to the bed, but could not elevate him up. He lay, straddled across the bed, where he had fallen. I got above him, put my hands underneath his arm pits and tried to pull. As thin as he was, I could not raise his body. BRUCE, WHY THE HELL AREN'T YOU HERE TO HELP ME? MICHAEL AND I NEED YOU. I NEED YOU. I CAN'T DO THIS ALONE, GOD. HELP, HELP, HELP.

"Michael, this is the nurse from Hell back again."
He wrinkled his face at me, in disapproval.
"Mike, I can't adjust your position to make you more comfortable. I know that you have to be up against the pillows to breath better. Please, Michael, can you move yourself?"
"Not yet, Ma. Don't worry. I'll be okay. I'm here. I'm home. Feels good. Thanks."

He closed his eyes, sighed, and looked perfectly contented. I wanted to scream with frustration. He lay in such an awkward manner across the bed, but I had to accept things as they were. I couldn't move him.

"I'll make you hot milk, Michael. Your stomach is empty."
"Okay, Mom. I love you. Good to be home."

I heated the milk, but he was deeply asleep when I got back. I left the milk, and turned out his light. When I think about it now, I should have woke him and ensured that he took additional fluid. By the time that I had scrubbed the bathroom and kitchen, everything suddenly crashed down on me. I have no reserve of strength left. I fell onto my bed and fell asleep.

CHAPTER TWO

Within an hour, the telephone woke me. I reached for the portable phone beside me, which David had provided. It was Anna.

"Is Michael home, Mom? Is he all right?"

"I'm sorry, Anna. I fell asleep. He's alive. He's very weak. His body has undergone a great deal of trauma from this experience. He's in his own bed, and that's important to Michael's emotional well-being. Anna, what happened at the doctor's today?

"Mom, I don't know. I waited for him, and took him home after he went to get his pills at the pharmacy. He kissed me and told me that he loved me, and we both had tears in our eyes. He walked away from me, and wouldn't answer the phone after that."

"Did you realize that he would take every pill he had hidden in this place? Did he tell you what he intended to do?"

"No, Mom, but I've had a terrible feeling in my stomach since six o'clock."

"Father calls that 'Motherly Instinct' stuff. When you love someone this much, I guess you feel their psychic vibrations. I've discovered that this bond between a mother and her child is more potent than I ever imagined."

Anna seemed to reach across the miles.

"Mom, I love you. Get some rest. I don't want you to get sick, too. You've been going hard, for so long. I don't know where you get your strength."

NOT A TOTAL WASTE

"I'm not strong, Anna. All that I do lately, is cry. Without control. The pain comes in waves, of its own accord. He's dying, Anna. We'll have him for just such a short time, now."

"I know that, Mom."

"I also feel badly about alienating Michael's friends. He needs ALL of his loyal friends, right now, while he still lives. They must think that I'm just a crazy, overbearing bitch."

"It's not your problem, Mom. You've done the best that you can. Please, just concentrate on Michael and your own health, now."

"Okay, dear. Anna, can you please come over tomorrow morning? I want to call Dr. Drake to make an appointment. I'm going to request morphine tablets for Michael. His pain must be alleviated. He doesn't complain, but he shouldn't have to take this torment. Not any longer."

"As soon as Sean and Jenni are off to school, I'll drive over."

It was nearly ten o'clock when Anna arrived Friday morning, and shortly before noon I entered the waiting room of Dr. Drake. He had agreed to see me between regularly scheduled patients. His specialty involved specifically tending AIDS patients. Seated in that room with me were several of these.

One was a young woman, in her early twenties, approximately six months pregnant. She was blond, with green eyes and a luminous dewy skin. AIDS can be transferred from an infected mother to an infant during pregnancy, delivery or during breast feeding. It is not an automatic sentence, however. Some babies are born free of the disease. On the other side of me, sat a young man in his late twenties or early thirties. He chatted with a woman who appeared to be his mother, planning a shopping trip to be completed after their appointment. The third patient seemed considerably older, was slightly built, wore thick-lensed glasses, and had thinning brown hair. However, upon closer examination, I recognized that he was more likely about Michael's age. A younger, slender man with shoulder-length black, shiny hair, wearing tight blue-jeans and T-shirt, with leather sandals on his bare feet, darted in. He picked up his prescription from the receptionist, chatted with her for a few moments, and then left. Whenever Dr. Drake picked up a patient's file from the receptionist he would look up, smile and greet any newcomer. He radiated empathy and kindness. This doctor had charisma.

He held the door for me when my turn arrived, and waved me towards a chair. I felt comfortable immediately, and knew why Michael felt safe with this doctor. I reached into my shopping bag and carefully unwrapped Michael's burgundy-coloured, knitted scarf from the sculpture. The Italian Binimi piece of Don Quixote was placed firmly on the centre of the desk. Dr. Drake looked bemused. Holding onto the edge of the chair for support, I explained,

"One of Michael's favourite classics is the story of Don Quixote. This is his Binimi sculpture, from Italy. Michael's too tired to fight windmills, anymore. He wanted you to have this, as a remembrance."

He put his head down, and swallowed hard, "How is Michael?"

"Not good. He took an overdose last night, but he vomited it into the sink. Some well-meaning friends called 911, so he was taken to the hospital. It was awkward getting him home, but thankfully a doctor recognized that he was terminally ill. His compassion permitted me to remove Michael from of the Emergency ward, instead of admitting him. He is back home now. His sister Anna is visiting with him."

"I see. Had he been stockpiling drugs for awhile?"

"He stated that he had saved some for over a year. He had also notified Dr. Baker that he intended to quit his medication, ten days ago. It was his decision, and as you know, he's a strong-willed young man."

"Yes, he is indeed. I swear that I don't know how he has kept alive this long. His weight yesterday was 100 lbs. Without his sister Anna to assist him, I am sure that he would not have come back to see me. Would you want to live under the "quality of life" conditions which he has been experiencing? I sure wouldn't. He can't eat anything, can't get out to be with his friends, and is suffering from so much pain--all of the time."

"Yes. His pain is especially bad at night. I guess that everything seems worse, at night. I am assuming that he came to say goodbye, and to pick up his prescription for a light sedative?"

"That's right. How can I help him, now?"

"Michael has previously refused morphine, because he demanded some functional control over his life conditions. We have discussed his steadily increasing pain level. He has agreed with me that he must accept small dosages of morphine, now."

NOT A TOTAL WASTE

"The average person, without Michael's veracity, would have been hospitalized. No way could they tolerate that intense suffering. That type of chronic pain is both destructive and demoralizing. He will require one tablet of morphine, every four hours."
"I'll administer these to him carefully."
"This additional drug will provide Michael with some relief from the severe cramping. He hurts to be touched or moved. It's obvious that his inability to swallow, the vomiting and pernicious diarrhea have impacted heavily upon his health. You realize that he is dying? That he has very little time remaining?"
"My mind admits that to be true. My emotions deny it. I still can't accept that he won't be with me, always. Maybe I'll never be able to accept that he is going to die."

Dr. Drake nodded, swallowed hard again and looked at the ceiling.

"Here are his prescriptions. Is there anything that you need for yourself?"
"Yes, doctor. I am in no state to take care of my students at this time. Would you please prepare a letter for my principal to verify that I am truly ill?"
"Without any doubt, you are incapacitated sufficiently that you would be no asset within a classroom. Your mind and soul are elsewhere. Emotional and physical exhaustion are defined as an illness. My secretary will provide you with a letter. Just give me a moment, and I'll explain to her what you require. Will this grant you permission to remain with Michael?"
"Yes, it will give me a legitimate sick leave."
"Will you require a prescription for a tranquilizer?"
"No, I don't want to take anything, if I can avoid it. I'm enervated, but I am afraid to sleep soundly, in case Michael needs me."
"All right...but...are you aware that you have additional responsibilities which you must attend to, now?"
"I'm not sure what you mean".
"Let me give this information to my secretary and I'll come back and outline those for you."

When he returned, Dr. Drake handed me paper and pen, and said,

"You had better write these things down. You will have to consider some funeral arrangements. Have you discussed Michael's wishes with him?"

"Yes. We've talked about it. Can you provide me with the name of an undertaker who is not homophobic? One that is situated close to Michael's apartment, and who will take care of his remains with dignity? Michael wants to be cremated, and he has mentioned the Rosar-Morrison Funeral Home on Sherbourne to me."

"They will not refuse to help you. You should go to them, after obtaining the prescription, and ask to see the Director. Go this afternoon. Be candid about Michael's AIDS, and his request to be cremated."

"When Michael dies, what should I do? His Living Will stipulates his desire to refuse any extra measures to extend his life. I've promised him. I am committed to supporting his request to die peacefully, in his own bed, in his own apartment. I want to be beside him, to hold him."

Both of our eyes filled.

"Contact me by telephone immediately. I have a beeper, so that my answering service will locate me. I will come to sign the death certificate. I have known Michael for over four years now, and his health has deteriorated drastically during the last three months."

"Yes."

"What about Michael's father? Michael and I have discussed that relationship."

"Bruce has supported Michael in every way that he can. It was never a "buddy-pal" support-system, but they have acquired a mutual respect. They have both tried to appreciate each other's virtues. What else can I say?"

"Michael said that he has not been in touch with his father for over two years."

"Many dysfunctional relationships are testy. I can't make excuses. Both Michael and I have felt a great deal of pain, because of the lack of communication with his father. Bruce just builds a high wall, and hides behind it. He's just not effective at showing affection."

"I see. Michael said that he and Anna were close."

"They've been good friends."

"You were the main care giver?"

"Well, I've had assistance from some of his devoted friends.

NOT A TOTAL WASTE

He has a few good, loyal and supportive pals. I feel really fortunate to have met some of them. Actually, I've grown to love them, too."

"How are Michael's finances?"

"Not lucrative. Far from it. He's run out of his unemployment funding. He has to apply to welfare, if he is going to live, but he knows that will be inadequate. He's been coping, with help from us. Michael has been existing on disability and a small insurance stipend since his earlier resignation. He's basically poverty-line. Maybe he doesn't look or sound like he should be poor. He's articulate, well-educated, and he dresses all right..."

"You must clarify that his income is restricted, when you talk to the Director at the funeral parlour. Social Services can provide some assistance for the costs of the cremation, and they can guide you towards that funding."

"I didn't know that."

"There will also be an application for death benefits. Ask the Director for his advice. He'll also arrange for additional copies of the death certificate. Once I have signed it, you must give it to the attendants when they remove Michael's remains. You can pick up the extra copies from the secretary at the funeral home, afterwards. You will require these, when you are tidying up his business affairs."

"I appreciate your help with this. I do have a Power of Attorney, and have promised Michael to take charge of those things. I didn't know which steps to take."

"You have his prescriptions. Your letter is ready for you at the front desk. Please call me as soon as you need me. For any reason. You can be very proud of Michael's courage. He is a brave young man. I have seldom seen such tenacity against the odds which he has faced."

I covered my eyes with my hands, and blew my nose. I must not break down here! There were patients in the outside office who must face this in their future, if no cure is found quickly enough. I owed it to them, and to Michael, to show the type of intestinal fortitude that he has steadily illustrated.

"Thank you, Dr. Drake, for helping Michael and me."

"He is a beautiful person. We will both miss him, very much."

I looked into his eyes and nodded. He reached over and patted me on the shoulder, and asked,

"Will you handle all of these details by yourself?"

"I must. There is no alternative."

"Michael often spoke of your strength, and of the loving relationship which you shared. He trusts and admires you. With your support, he can have a small measure of control, until the end. He is badly atrophied and dehydrated. I must warn you--the morphine may cause him to hallucinate, and to drift sleepily. The diarrhea will cease, as his body functions slow down. This is natural. Don't let these things alarm you. Take care of yourself, too. Michael would want that."

I couldn't respond, but simply nodded, let myself out of his office and picked up the letter from the receptionist.

Over a cup of tea, and many Kleenex tissues later, the Director of the funeral home helped me to complete the forms and detailed arrangements, related to Michael's death and cremation. With the monies I had withdrawn from Michael's small bank account, I paid for a square brass urn. I asked that it be engraved with his name, the date of his birth, and when the time came--the date of his death. It had an engraved cross on one side, but was otherwise unadorned. It had a simple refinement in its design. Michael would have approved of its restraint and quiet elegance. With the documents provided to me, I went to the Social Services to obtain funding assistance for the cremation costs. Those documents were signed, and returned to the funeral home. Finally, I filled Michael's prescriptions. By four o'clock, I stumbled home, feeling just pooped, to Michael.

Anna had prepared tea, and Michael sat propped in his bed, wide awake.

"I have your medication from Dr. Drake, Mike. He appreciated getting the sculpture. He's going to keep it on the desk in his office."

"Oh, good!" Michael beamed. "I liked that piece. It was a great gift idea, since Dr. Drake is another artsy-type. He'd find pleasure in its sleek lines and obvious humour."

I smiled back at Michael, amazed at the continual lucidity of his mind. What a bizarre type of hell this was, to have such brilliance encased within a disintegrating body. It was so unfair.

NOT A TOTAL WASTE

"Well, Michael, what can I get for you to drink? Will you have lemonade or iced tea with your morphine tablet?"
"Lemonade sounds good, Mom. Thanks for seeing Dr. Drake for me."
"I loved him. He reminds me of a typical '60's flower child, all grown up. He dresses in a comfortable fashion, even down to his leather sandals and manicured beard. He's really a kind man, son. He thinks the world of you, too, dear. Its apparent that you're both good friends."
"Yes, he's special. Mom, has Anna gone? Please Mom, may I have all of those morphine tablets and whatever else I can find?"
"Michael, don't say that. NO."
"Please, Mom. I love you. But I do want to take them all, right now. Mom, I WANT TO DIE."

Michael sat up straight and looked directly into my eyes. I stepped back, and leaned limply against his bedroom door. The stress from the doctor's office, funeral parlour and Social Service appointments seemed to have piled up on me. I felt vulnerable, and weepy. How could I ever deal with the stark reality of Michael's desire for death?

"Michael, don't do this. Please. Behave yourself. I'm going to keep these tablets hidden from you. Anna has not gone. I'm certain that she will have heard you. You won't want to upset her."
"Oh, God, Mom. I've had all the suffering that I need. The dream is over, Mom. No miracles. It's done. Just let me go."

My hands shook as I handed him one tablet with his lemonade. He took it, sighed, and leaned back against the pillows. He turned his face resolutely away from me, towards his bookcases.

CHAPTER THREE

Within moments, Corey unlocked the apartment door with his own key and walked jauntily towards me, as I stood outside of Michael's bedroom. Smiling, he stood with his hands on his hips and peered into Michael's room.

"Hi, Mike. How're you doing?"
"Not good. Mom went to see Dr. Drake and got morphine for me. It took her damn near four hours! She just gave me one, now. Do you want some iced tea?"
"Sure. After that, you're getting dressed and we're going for a ride to the Beaches."
"What?" I asked, and stared in disbelief at Corey.
"Don't worry. This is between Mike and me. I'll take good care of him. It's warmer today. We'll take a little stroll along the sandy beach. The sunshine and fresh air will do him good."
Michael smiled up at Corey, and said, "OKAY!"

While I handed Corey his iced tea, I wondered how on earth he could take Michael for a drive in his car. Michael was incapacitated and skeletal. He looked too ill to move.

"Mom, can you look in the drawer for my bathing suit and green GAP T-shirt? I want to wear that today."
"Son, it's not that warm. You'd be better off with your jeans, or your knee-length shorts."

NOT A TOTAL WASTE

"My bathing suit, Ma. It's what I want." He boldly contracted his brows in displeasure to register his famous scowl, so I obediently located his bathing suit.

"Here, Michael. You might also want to take this bath towel to sit on, so that your back will be cushioned and more comfortable."

"I'll help him. Come on, Mike. Let's get your little ass into this bathing suit."

"I hope it won't fall off me. I've lost a bit of weight."

"Your butt was always small, anyway. That's why the girls pinched it."

"That's been awhile. Nothing left to pinch, now."

"Who cares? It'll be just you and me and the Beaches."

They were gone quickly, and the silence seemed magnified. Anna sauntered in slowly from the kitchen.

"That was interesting. Sure hope that Corey has an air-conditioned car. If Mike loses his bowel control, it could get nasty."

"Yetch. Well, no matter. Corey can handle anything. He has cleaned up after Michael during previous visits."

"Yeh? That's what good friends are for, I 'spose."

"You should have seen the effect that Corey had over Michael in the hospital. He and Ted could get him to eat, when I had given up. It was amazing. He'd even finish his vegetable soup."

"I guess friendship and love are close commodities, Mom."

"They also share mischief and fun."

They were gone for three hours. The Beaches was another interesting residential section of Toronto. When I was a child, it had been considered a summer resort neighbourhood, connected to the central core of the city by an electric railroad. The rapidly expanding population had engulfed the little summer cottages, and most of those had now become converted permanent homes. During World War II, my mother and aunt Martha used to take us to swim beside the most notable landmark of the Beaches--the Boardwalk. For more than two miles, it stretched along Lake Ontario. From Queen Street East between the Greenwood Racetrack and Neville Park, the area now was crowded with various stores, pubs and restaurants. Anna and I had been there to see a psychic at a tea room one sunny afternoon, earlier in the year. I could see why Corey wanted to take Michael for a drive along the Boardwalk. That area of the Beaches was a pleasant spot for a stroll on a sunny afternoon, and it would give them some privacy to chat.

After Anna drove back to Hamilton, I lay down and closed my eyes. I didn't sleep, because so many thoughts tugged at my subconscious. I took a short walk down to Gerrard Street to pick up some fresh juices and cucumber for Michael, and some sandwich fixings--in case Corey decided to stay for a snack. I also picked up a newspaper, hoping to help myself nod off and nap. It had debilitated me, planning Michael's cremation. Yet, there he was, off with Corey to the Beaches. However, I felt confident that Corey would protect him and bring him back safely.

When they returned, they removed their canvas-topped running shoes at the door. They were literally filled with sand, and soaking wet.

"Naughty boys. Now I'll have to throw both pairs into the laundromat washers."

Michael did not look at me, but headed straight to his bedroom. Corey grinned sadly, and then followed him down the hall.

"Do you have anything to drink for Mike and me? Some of that lemonade or O.J. would be nice."

They sat drinking their juice and chatting quietly. They were both subdued and weary. I went back to the front room to permit them their privacy. On his way out, Corey asked,

"Does Mike own a pair of sandals that I could borrow? My shoes are drenched, too."
"Of course. He has those leather BIRKENSTOCK sandals that I bought for him when he was in the hospital. They just fall off his feet, now. His weight loss has even affected his shoe size. You could use them, I think."
"They'll fit. We both wear the same shoe size. Mind if I borrow them?"
"Help yourself. Do you want me to wash your shoes when I wash Michael's?"

NOT A TOTAL WASTE

"No, that won't be necessary. I'll take care of that. Thanks. I'll be over tomorrow to see Mike."

After Corey left, I tried again to contact David. I had left a message on his answering machine related to Michael's hospitalization, and this time I explained that he was now taking morphine for pain relief. It was unlike David not to return my calls. However, we were each dealing with our pain in our own ways. I also called Bruce to let him know of Michael's change in medication.

It was not until after Michael's death that Corey explained to me that while at the Beaches, Michael had submerged himself in Lake Ontario. He had tried to drown himself. Corey had carried him out, and they had discussed the impact that his potential death, by suffocation in the water, could have had upon me. Michael knew that my father and uncle had died in that manner, during a fishing trip near Prince Albert. Michael told Corey that he had reconsidered and was grateful that Corey had rescued him. Perhaps the combination of morphine and tortuous pain prompted Michael's actions. The experience saddened them, and made Corey fully aware of Michael's death wish.

Michael had not indicated suicidal tendencies until the pain grew burdensome. He had always been able to count his blessings, no matter what problems he faced. Joy and exuberance are apparent in the following letter, written to me in November, 1989. He had resigned from his chosen teaching career that month, and I was concerned that he would be suffering depression. His health prognosis did not, however, represent a death knell to him.

Chere Maman,

Ici moi. Yes, I actually have time to write. It is a glorious, cool, sunny fall day after an early morning rain. My 'huistput' (sp?) is cooling in the blue and white Delft bowl that you gave me. I can actually put it in my mouth without scalding it. Cubed steak, beets, beet greens, carrots, baby potatoes, celery, leeks and onions cooked in a big pot with lots of beef broth, thyme, sage and salt. OISHI DESU. Perfect for the day.

I have torn up the rotten part of the bathroom floor and filled it in with parquet tiles bought on the cheap and auto body filler (a really gross pinkish colour) which I have spent a day sanding. Penny has been bitching because I have dirtied her bathroom just after she had cleaned it and because everything tastes like fibreglass (the body filler has fibreglass fibres in it). No joy at all that she will not have to trod on rusty old nails or fall through a crumbling floor or tear her nylons or feet on a piece of tile. "I wear slippers", she says. Hmmph! At any rate, all the slopping and levelling and gluing and sanding and painting are making for a beautifully restful time pour moi.

The 'huistput' is consumed, I have washed my dark load and it is presently drying in my funky new little washer/dryer (plastic, made by I.T.T. in Belgium, only does 4.5 lbs. at a time), and the sky has darkened. When I finish tapping this letter off to you, I shall return to my mystery novel and sneak under the sheets with a hot tea and cookies. There are some pleasures in being ill.

David took me out for dinner twice this week. He is being very good, and spoiling me. I had to tell him of my AIDS, of course, since he would need to know my reason for my leaving teaching. We ran into Ted at Boots after dinner. Ted was maudlin as hell. He has had two friends die on him with AIDS in the past month, and he is also nervous about turning thirty. He is terrified that I will 'up and pop off' on him, as he made very obvious last night. I explained that I am not about to pop off, that quitting teaching was a sure signal of my determination to protect my health above and beyond anything, and that he should STOP worrying about me. Silly boy. Of course, there is also the fact that Ted was smashed out of his tree, which can be fun...(on occasion).

I am having dinner with Ted at a Japanese place in the Big Carrot Mall on the Danforth at eight tonight. I shall have tempura soba (they have the best soba - made in Vancouver, but better than any I ever had in Japan) and slurp my noodles noisily. Ted will probably have the bento again. I think I shall avoid the sake. I had a martini and a calvados last night, so I think that is quite enough for me for a week, considering that I had a similar amount on Tuesday when I went out with David and Val (a gorgeous actor friend of David's who I would kill for). The restaurant on Tuesday was appalling - one of the items on the menu was called 'escargots

NOT A TOTAL WASTE — 189

tropicana' and consisted of snails, papaya and banana!!!!! BERK!!! I settled on the filet with frites. What can they do to filet with frites? They can make the frites out of sweet potato, is what they can do. AAAGHGHGHGH!

Le Souffle last night was much nicer - simple Lobster bisque followed by a four-cheese souffle, a decent bottle of burgundy, and absolutely wonderful service. She got a humungous tip. I like Le Souffle - it's friendly. Have you noticed how much I've been talking about food in this letter? You worry about my appetite, Chere Maman. See, I AM eating.

Lucy is travelling in Italy. Penny and I are looking forward to her return in the spring. Eagerly. She has been to some places where I have not travelled, and I'm jealous. I yearn to be there too, especially at this time of the year. I have never been to San Gimignanao, but I have been to Firenze, Paestum (there is a nice beach there, too) Napoli, Sorrento, Assissi and Sienna. I loved Sienna in the summer--I got to watch the running of the Paglio, the most famous horse race on the continent, which takes place in the central square. Summer in Sienna does have many compensations. Milan was one place that I didn't stay - no real desire. Amalfi I still have not done, but the Amalfi coast is nevertheless where I want to retire. I hope that my health will hold that long! There is a restaurant that I have heard of in Ravello, and a hotel, too...I love Italy. Shame that Lucy was robbed so often.

But enough drivel. I do want to give you some other news. The school board has agreed to give me four weeks of sick leave, so that I am now officially entitled to 29.3% of my salary. I sure hate to be on the poverty-line.

I am waiting for a call from Teletron re a telephone answering and computer linkage job, and have mailed in many other applications for a part-time type of sedentary occupation. Have to retain that structure in my life. I will be O.K. (far from rich, but O.K.). Maybe I'll play bicycle courier come spring - a fabulous $50/day but good exercise...Na! No way! What is a reasonably intelligent, capable individual with lousy health to do to make money? Forward any ideas, please, Maman.

Well, I guess that's really all that I have to say, except that I'm back up to 150 lbs (from 143) and feel much happier. Hope you are doing well, too (gosh, the first lines about someone other than myself). Don't worry, Ma. I'm going to beat this disease.

LOVE AND KISSES, Michael.

CHAPTER FOUR

That evening, after Michael had eaten some baked brown beans and finished half a glass of milk, he asked if we could rent the video film STAR TREK V. I scurried down to the corner store and selected it and four others. I thought that he might become restless and want to view different ones, later. He watched the movie for about three-quarters of an hour and then turned away from me. He snuggled into the fetal position and appeared as though he might sleep.

"Want me to turn this off, Michael, so that you can grab some shut eye?"

"That would be very nice. I'm really tired, Ma."

"No problem. I'm in the same state. Sleep well. Don't hesitate to call out if you need anything, Michael."

"Ma?"

"What, Mike?"

"Would you like to wrap one of my P.D. James mysteries for Dad, for Father's Day? Because..."

"Michael, I wrapped that Michener's book on the Caribbean, after you said that you were finished with it. I don't how how the hell you read that thing, because it was so big--and the print was so small. How did your eyes manage?"

"I just plodded along. There was some good historical stuff in it. His writing indicates a superb eye for landscapes--architectural, human and geographical. My vision isn't what it used to be, though. It's getting worse daily. Like everything else."

"I can't sit still long enough for him to finish with his descriptive sections. Guess I'm not left-brained enough. Father reads with his atlas beside him, to verify the location of each single place that Michener mentions."

"Yes, he always liked that author. Analytical thinking, maybe."

"Too tedious for me. Takes concentration that I don't possess, lately."

"Now Mother, not really tedious. More like...kind of ponderous...sometimes. But, are you still consuming about the usual number of books, magazines and newspapers?"

"Mmmhmm. Plus the texts needed for curriculum research. Good thing I learned to speedread when I was twenty."

"You wear me out just thinking of it, Mom."

"Guess that I'll burn out, before I rust out."

"Get some sleep, Ma. Thanks for taking care of the book for Father. Just wrap it. It won't need a card. Tell him that it's from my library, though. Good choice, actually, since he really likes Michener."

"Okay. I'll make sure of it. God bless, son."

Because Michael's eyesight was failing, he had difficulty reading small print, and tired quickly watching the television. He fell asleep fairly fast, probably due to the morphine tablet and the one sleeping pill which he had requested. He'd had quite a day and badly needed to rest. I took care of the few dishes and straightened the kitchen. After a warm bath, I went to bed and slept soundly.

Anna returned around ten o'clock the following morning. She sat with Michael, while I did the laundry and shopped for groceries. When I returned, Michael was awake and ready for his fortified milk shake. While he sipped that, he looked carefully at me and blurted out,

"Mom, please call Bob."

"Why, dear? It's Saturday, and he'll be really busy."

"Mom, you have to have your hair cut. It looks like 'Scissorhand' or some mad designer was at it. Who cut it last time?"

"You remember--it was a mistake. But I'm certain that Bob won't be able to fit me in, Michael."

NOT A TOTAL WASTE

"Try. Tell him I asked him to see what he could do, and that I'm ill. If he can't do it, call Tom. He's a good friend to Kim and David. Check Bob first."

Michael had introduced me to Bob, one of Toronto's outstanding hairstylists, at least ten years ago. I had followed him from one establishment to the next, because no-one could give me the type of styling he offered. He usually cut my hair once or twice a year when I managed to get to Toronto for conferences. Since Michael's sickness, I was frequently in the city, but had little time to make a hair stylist appointment. Now, it bothered Michael that my hair was not "up to par". When I called Bob, I explained Michael's request and he managed to find room for me at 1:30 that afternoon.

"How is Michael doing?"

"Not good, Bob. I'm afraid that it won't be long."

"I'm sorry! Let's see if we can fix this cut, so that he'll be satisfied, too."

At two o'clock, my hair had been washed, cut, but not yet blown dry. Suddenly, I had an all-consuming feeling of rising panic and excused myself from Bob. I had to call Anna to allay the terror that I felt.

"Anna, it's Mom. Please tell me the truth. Is Michael alive? Is he in trouble? I have this awful feeling."

"Mom, get your hair cut. Michael wants you to do that. He's hallucinating and sees little yellow ducks everywhere. He collapsed in the bathroom, Mom, and fell on the floor. I picked him up and placed him on the toilet. Now he's back in bed."

"Anna, I'm going to just come home. I can't stand being away from Michael right now. Who cares how I look? I just want to be with him. I feel as if I'm going to have a damned anxiety attack, or something."

"No, Mom. Michael sent you to get your hair fixed. You can't handle it the way it was cut before, and Michael wants you to look your best. Do it HIS way."

"Is he awake?"

"He's just resting. His eyes are closed, but he's not asleep. He just asked, 'Where's my Mom?' and I reminded him about the hair appointment. He said, 'Okay,' and now he's just waiting for you. Finish it up and get back, Mom. See you soon."

I explained to Bob what was happening and he quickly finished my hair for me. As I rose to leave, he hugged me and then handed me a large, multi-coloured bouquet of flowers for Michael. It was a beautiful, cheerful spray of spring flowers, tied with a large blue ribbon and covered with clear, crisp lucite.

"There you are--no, no payment accepted. The hair cut is on the house, for Michael. Give him the flowers and tell him that I love him. Take care of yourself, too. Here's my card with my personal number on it--please leave me a message about Michael. Let me know how he's doing. Come and see me when you get to Toronto, later. Promise?"

I burbled thank you's, nodded and ran. A taxi took me home quickly. I was back home by three forty-five. Michael was awake when I entered his room. Nervously, I blithered,

"Look, dear, at this profusion of beautiful flowers. Bob sent them for you. They're every colour of the rainbow. Have you ever seen such a collection? Aren't they lovely?"
"Yes, but turn around. I want to see your hair."
"Is it all right?"
"That's much better, Mother. Much better. Promise that you'll go back to Bob later, Ma. And that you won't put that dark-brown rinse on your hair, anymore."
"Okay. No more 'kitchen beautician'. I promise."
"Use light golden brown, Mom. The grey will be lighter, then, and the rest will stay dark. It'll be softer for you. Not so harsh."
"All right, Michael."
"Mom, the traffic will be picking up on the Queen Elizabeth and the 401. I'll have to get going. Michael, can I give you a kiss?"
"No. But you can kiss my cheek."

Michael and Anna hugged, kissed cheeks, and I took her to the door.

"Mom, he had more hallucinations. Those damn yellow ducks. Everywhere."
"It's the morphine, dear. You drive home safely, now."
"Will you call me later, please, Mom? Let me know how Mike is?"
"Yes, dear. I will. Watch the traffic carefully."

NOT A TOTAL WASTE

"Can you call me after six o'clock?"
"Of course. Now, just get going home. Don't worry. I'll take good care of Michael. Love you."

She nodded, turned and was gone out of the door so quickly that it seemed as though she had evaporated. I blinked, but she did not reappear. I returned to Michael's darkened room. He lay, propped up on his pillows, looking at me quizzically.

"Mom? Could you please turn on the television? Do you know what's on?"
"Nothing but World of Sports, and things like that."
"Well, put on Father's boring sports. The narrator's voice will drone on and relax me."
"Are you teasing? You've always hated watching sporting events. Do you want to go right to sleep?"
"Somehow, it reminds me of Father and a typical Saturday at home. I'd find that comforting right now."
"Oh, okay, dear. Oh, Michael, I've just found the five videos that I rented last night. They'll have to be returned, or they'll charge me double. It will take me just a few minutes to run them down to the corner."
"Sure, Mom. I'd like some carbonated lemon water to sip, though, please, before you go. And Mom...you know the cash that you always leave for me, on top of my dresser?"
"Do you mean the emergency money?"
"Right. Will you put it in an envelope and seal it?"
"Now?"
"Just do it, Mom. Write Corey's name on it. Save it for him, for later. He can't work full-time, anymore."
"Done. I will give it to him...later."

I took Michael his lemon water and then dashed, like a marathon runner, to return the videos to the little store on Sherbourne Street. I literally tossed the cassettes onto the counter, nodded at the kindly, oriental proprietor and rushed out of the door. I darted in and around traffic and back down Berkley Street to Michael. When I returned, out of breath and panting like a dog in the middle of August, Michael had completed his drink. He was leaning against his pillows, watching the televised sports program.

"Hi, Son," I puffed. "What can I get for you?"

"Nothing, Mom. You sure got back fast. Please lie down here, beside me."

"Oh yetch, and listen to the crummy sports? I never was much of a jock. Good thing we don't have to drink beer and eat hot dogs."

"Now, Mom, the voice IS kind of soothing."

"Well, I guess that you're trying to recapture that Saturday afternoon feeling, as if Father were here."

"Yeh. Maybe that's it. I seem to need that, right now. And Ma...something else. Did you get in touch with Lucy? I asked you to phone her, didn't I?"

"I tried to call Lucy, Mike. Usually she has he answering machine on, but this time it simply rang and rang. Either she is not answering, or not home. She might be using a machine that screens the return number of the person calling. She was pretty mad at me."

"She is special, Mom. Very special to me. She and Therese may have gone to Montreal for the week-end. Please keep on calling her later, until you reach her. Tell her thanks for getting me to the hospital. That I'm sorry..."

"Okay, I will. Michael, I'm sorry too. Lucy and I just lit into each other. I guess that I WAS irrational. We both love you. We were both trying to help you, in different ways. She may forgive me, eventually. I remember how close you have been, over the years. Only five years ago you both spoke of marriage, and having your own home. You were going to experience that 'traditional family life'...remember? You wanted to escape the penalties of the gay scene. She wanted to travel with you, too, and you talked of children. I know of three gay men who have families."

"That was before the positive blood test wrecked up everything, Mom. I would never have risked hurting Lucy in any way. That was pre-BIG A."

"BIG A. They used to whisper about cancer as being the BIG C. Another medical bogeyman."

"Now its only the person with AIDS that terrifies people, Mom. They're still ignorant about the disease. Anyway, about Lucy. Let's not dwell on 'what might have been'. Just remember to call her." He sounded agitated, and deeply fatigued.

"Of course I'll call her. Maybe later I'll take her and Therese to Thai Magic for dinner, the way you planned. Good idea?"

"Excellent idea. Sorry I couldn't do it, Mom." He sounded weary, but articulated carefully, as if with effort.

"You're right about the Big A, Michael. You know that I've had cancer, yet I don't inform people about that, either."
"Better not to, Ma. It scares and repels them."
"You're right. You've experienced enough of that 'How long are you going to be around, dearie?' look."
"Yeh. Women who have survived breast cancer get the most gawks. People play mental games about how deformed the breasts must appear."
"That's just so gross. It's as disgusting as those creepy men who make the "Can I watch?" comments to lesbian couples."
"Ummm. It's that minority hatred again...females, homosexuals, racial discrimination." His voice was muffled, and his answers were slower. He was all in, yet he continued speaking softly,
"Nothing new, Mom. No miracles yet."
"I guess that the big C and the big A have a lot in common, Mike. No quick fix expected for viral diseases. Anyway, on that cheerful note--would you like me to get your plush puppy and teddy bear, to join our sports bash?"
"No way. Hmmph! Leave those guys. Let them burn their asses on the heat register." His anger surprised me.
"Not today, Mike. It's June. No heat's turned on."
"Right. No wonder I'm so damned cold."
"Can I get you another blanket, Michael? Do you want something hot to drink?"
"No, Ma. Just stay here...beside me." His smile was gentle, and his eyes showed tenderness.

Within ten minutes, Michael had pushed his pillows aside, rolled over and stretched out onto his stomach. His left hand was tucked underneath his neck and tugged his blanket closely around his shoulders. He splayed his legs wide, with his right foot bent slightly, pushing hard against the firm mattress. Michael's right arm was close to me and I patted it lovingly. After a few moments, I just rested my hand on his arm, as lightly as possible. His face was turned away from me and he began to be drift off to sleep. Softly, gently, I heard his voice say,

"Don't leave, Mom. I love you."
"I love you so much, Michael. And I'm very proud of you." My throat was constricted with emotion as I choked out those few words.

In less than two minutes, the television stand, which we had built together, collapsed like a house of cards. The television, VCR, air filter machine, the few videos which he owned and the shelving, all went flying.

"Oh, no! No matter, Michael, I'll just put the television on this little side table."

"Okay, Mom. Sorry about the stand." His voice sounded distant and strained.

"It doesn't matter, son. We had trouble building it, anyway. I'll give the pieces to Corey and he can fix it for himself. He's good at that."

"Okay, Ma. That's fine with me. He likes IKEA."

"Everything is tidied up, dear. May I still stay beside you, here?"

"Please, Mom. Don't go. Because...it get's lonely, when you're gone. Just stay." He snuggled against his pillows, and pulled his blankets closer to his neck to keep warm.

I checked the clock radio beside Michael's bed, and saw that it was five o'clock. The sports programming would persist until six. I turned the volume on the television down a bit, and left his bedside lamp turned on. I wriggled closer to Michael to help him to retain body heat, rested my hand gently on his right arm, and closed my eyes.

Within fifteen minutes, Michael's breathing became raspy, but maintained a steady rhythm. Noises emanating from his lungs distressed me. I hoped that the morphine tablet reduced some of his torture. I couldn't seem to settle down after that, but lay beside him. Feeling nervous and restless, I worried that my inner turmoil might upset Michael. I propped a pillow under my neck and looked at the television screen, without really watching the program. The film inside my mind rolled pictures from the past, which I saw with intensive detail.

By 5:30, Michael's breathing changed drastically. It was more shallow, with extended time lapses between each breath. It did not seem to be laboured, but it had altered enough for me to sit up and listen. I leaned closer and squinted directly into Michael's face. His countenance was relaxed, eyes closed and he breathed through his partially opened mouth. He slept deeply. His pulse had slowed. My

NOT A TOTAL WASTE

heart skipped and I sat rigidly still. I listened intently to Michael's breathing. As I shifted closer towards him, I noticed that it had become harder to hear each breath. I was getting frightened. First, there would be a breath and then there would be quiet, without a breath. Then, softly, Michael would breathe again. What was happening? Was this it? OH NO, GOD. Not now. NOT NOW. PLEASE--LET ME HAVE HIM A LITTLE LONGER. PLEASE, GOD.

Tears filled my eyes. Michael was leaving me. I knew it. He was drifting away from me. I must remain very quiet and still. He must not be disturbed, or bothered. For some reason, I thought it was important for Michael, that everything remain calm and peaceful. I must not cry out, or weep aloud. He must not be upset, or held back. The atmosphere must be serene to help him pass over. I don't know why I thought that way, but it seemed true somehow.

THANK YOU GOD...THAT I AM HERE...BESIDE HIM. HE TRAVELLED SO MUCH, GOD, THAT HE COULD HAVE BEEN HALF-WAY AROUND THE WORLD--AND DIED ALONE. I'M GRATEFUL, BUT STILL--I'M SCARED, GOD. MY SON HAS NEVER DIED BEFORE, AND I DON'T KNOW WHAT TO DO. HOW CAN I HELP HIM? LET ME BE STRONG, GOD, AND LET HIM GO QUIETLY, GENTLY INTO THE NIGHT. I stayed very still with my hand upon his arm. It felt welded there, as if it was an essential part of him. Carefully, I reached across his inert body and picked up the phone. I pushed the blue button, with my thumb.

"Hello, Mom?"
"Yes, it's me, dear. Michael's breathing has changed. He's unconscious, Anna. The doctor warned me that his body functions would slow down, because he is severely dehydrated from the vomiting and diarrhea."
"Mom, what are you telling me?"
"Michael is leaving us, dear. Please pray for him."
"I have been, Mom. And I've asked for help for him."
"I can't talk, Anna. Just pray hard."
"I will. Call me back, Mom. Please."
"Right. Pray now."

The tears flowed down my face, and I sniffled involuntarily. I prayed for renewal for Mike and strength for his loved ones. Then, I pushed the red button to call Bruce. He picked up the phone on the first ring.

"Hello?"

"Michael is dying, Bruce. Please, pray hard for him."

"Oh. Where is he?" His voice seemed to echo in a vacant chamber.

"Here, in his apartment. Beside me. In his own bed."

"The way that he wanted."

"Yes." I choked and blew my nose.

"Did you check with his doctor?"

"Yesterday. Nothing can help him. He's gone into a coma. He's sleeping deeply and breathing strangely. Please, just pray for him."

"Yes...call me...later", he mumbled.

"Right."

I replaced the telephone quietly. Then, I tried to call Lucy one more time, without success. I tried David, but there was no answer. I decided to contact Corey and Ted later, when I felt stronger. There was no-one else to call, to beg for prayers. Only family mattered, now. Some things have to be done alone.

THANK YOU GOD, FOR LETTING ME GIVE BIRTH TO MICHAEL, AND FOR PLACING ME CLOSE TO HIM, WHEN HE MUST DIE. I listened to his gentle, irregular breathing, and lightly kissed his cheek. My prayers became silent, steady intercessions on Michael's behalf. I begged for his deliverance from his interminable pain. I pleaded for relief from his anguished loneliness. I prayed for the gift of peace for Michael, a peace not available to him on this earth.

At ten minutes after six, that Saturday June 8th, 1991 Michael died. He breathed five or six short, quick, sharp gasps. I kept my right hand on his arm, but rapidly moved my left hand to press my fingers against the notch in Michael's jawbone, about one inch in front of the angle of his jaw. I knew where the pressure points were located, from the First Aid courses I had taken. I searched carefully for a pulse. I could not locate one. Michael did not breath again. I took his wrist, pressed for the pulse, but found none. Michael was gone.

NOT A TOTAL WASTE

I patted him lovingly, slipped off the bed and onto my knees. I bowed my head, prayed and wept. With my eyes closed, I reached my hands upwards towards the ceiling, and offered my only dear son, weeping copiously.

"Take my Michael, please God. Take him from this hell, this testing place, into your arms. Take care of him for me, Mother Mary. Please ask your own sweet son, Jesus, to take care of my Michael. Cherish him, God. Keep him safe. Please help him. Please."

I sat back on the edge of Michael's bed, rocking myself, weeping and moaning in anguished grief. For some reason, I looked upwards and stared in wide-eyed disbelief. Closely aligned against the ceiling, on the wall which had the window and his bookcases, there stretched a golden, pinkish glow. It seemed to be a luminous, golden fog. My tears stopped and I sat in awe. As I watched, this warm, amber cloud began to slowly dissipate, as if scattered by a genial, temperate breeze. Was this an hallucination? Why did it provide me with such a powerful warmth, a sensation of intense love and wisdom? Now, I experienced complete calmness and a measure of control. Dry-eyed, I stopped trembling. Where did these responses come from? Why was it that I no longer needed to weep? Instead, I felt joy and elation. Was this only a figment of my imagination?

Then, I noticed that the illuminated digits, which indicated the time on Michael's electric clock-radio, were pulsing and fluctuating wildly. There must have been either a power surge, or shortage. When? What had caused it? Initially, I was frightened. Then, I remembered that the wobbly television stand had collapsed and that the electrical connections were inadequate in this apartment. Probably, the clock was plugged into the same area as the television, VCR, heater and air filter. When they were affected, perhaps the clock-radio was, too. There had to be some rational explanation.

I returned to bed and cuddled closer to Michael's body, needing to be near him. I felt a maternal desire to protect him. Instinctively, I put my arm across his shoulder. Something in my subconscious reminded me that there was nothing to fear for Michael, any longer. In a matter of moments, I felt enormous relief. Michael was out of pain. He would never hurt, again. He would never feel rejected or lonely. THANK YOU, GOD. TAKE CARE OF HIM FOR ME. PLEASE.

Despite my loss of Michael, I felt that this release was the right thing for him. I was submerged within a sensation of peacefulness and composure. I lay beside his body, with my hand on his bare shoulder, feeling Michael's warmth slowly ebb. His hands grew cold first and then, his feet. His chest retained his body warmth longer. Because he lay on his tummy, the small of his back stayed warm the longest. I rested my hand there. I spoke to Michael with love, as if he could still hear me. I was grateful for having shared his precious life.

The jubilance which I experienced during those first few hours, never recurred. Initially, it was replaced by a numbness, by a shock so stultifying that I could scarcely function. Later, my body was hit hard by a crushing anguish that throbbed and racked my body with pain. In a cyclical fashion, those feelings moved in alternating patterns, without restraint. Emotions held sway over me, gripping and twisting me in torment. I tried, vainly, to intellectualize them to a state of oblivion. This was my grief.

I stayed beside Michael, resting my hand on his cooling body for half an hour. My mind raced through his lifetime. Then I reached for the phone. I called Bruce first and then phoned Anna. Afterwards, I telephoned Dr. Drake's office. He was not available, but the answering service promised to notify him. Snuggled securely against Michael, I waited for that return call. At twenty to seven, Corey called.

"Hi, Maria. Could I please talk to Michael?"
"I'm sorry, Corey. He's gone. He died at 6:10."
"I'm coming right over."
"Okay."

I opened the door to let Corey into the apartment. We hugged each other tightly, for comfort. He went directly to the bedroom.

"May I please be alone with Mike, for a few minutes?"
"Certainly, Corey."

I waited in the dining room, on the black futon near the window. When Corey came out, I looked up and said,

NOT A TOTAL WASTE

"He simply went to sleep, Corey. The television stand fell apart, just before he died. He wanted you to take it, put it back together, and keep it."

"I could do that. I have a friend who works at the factory where Mike bought it. If there are any parts missing, he could get them for me."

"Good idea. You know, I think that Mike intended it for you, from the first day that he bought it."

"There are a few things of Mike's that I would like to have, to remember him."

"Oh, Corey...of course. They might help you to feel closer to him. You decide what would mean the most to you."

"May I have his new shoes? The ones with the buckles? They would fit me."

"That's right. You wear the same size. Try them on."

Initially, my feelings had been confused. I had exerienced both sadness and delight that Corey would wear those buckled shoes. Those were the shoes that had been Michael's pride and joy, that had taken us four different taxi trips to locate. I had polished them for him three times, until they shone and sparkled. Now, they looked strangely different upon Corey's feet. Almost immediately, I experienced a feeling of rapture rush over me. It was perfect. They'd really be enjoyed and those shoes would provide Corey with many happy memories of Mike. Magic shoes. Not Dorothy's red slippers, exactly. Now, Corey would wear them, use them, walk in them, and play.

"Oh yes, Corey. NOW those shoes will dance! Right?"

He grinned at me, his eyes sparkling with unshed tears, and he replied,

"Yes. That's right. They'll dance."

"Make sure that they do, dear. Often. It will be as though Michael is sharing the dancing and fun, with you."

"May I ask for his knapsack? The black one that is hanging there? Mike always used it when we went biking together. Somehow, I imagine it still on his back as he rode in front of me. If you don't mind, I would love to have it."

"Then you ought to have it, Corey. Aren't there other things that have special memories for you? Please don't be bashful to ask for them now, before they are packed or discarded."

"Well, there is one thing," he said softly. "It's the print on the dining room wall, over near Mike's stereo equipment. Mike and I talked about it, often."

"No problem. I don't remember it. Can we go and look at it, and take it down for you?"

We walked down the long hallway, into the dining room.

"Oh, now I remember it. That colourful, humerous print from the Paris art show. Corey, Mike mentioned to me last April that he thought you might enjoy it. Please help yourself, since you can reach it better than I. Did you bring your car? You should take these few things, along car."

"I appreciate having these, very much. I hesitated asking for them at first, because I was afraid you might think that I was being mercenary. Mike was an important part of my life. I'm sure that Anna will want to keep many of Mike's things to feel close to him, too."

"Michael wanted her to have them, Corey. His will leaves everything to me, but we verified his wishes before his death. I will have his artwork framed. Some day Anna and the children will want to reminisce over those pieces. I am not sure about his stereo equipment and the computer. He wanted me to use those. However, maybe Anna might require them for the children, Jenni and Sean. I'm just not sure. There's lots of time to decide. I'll talk it over with Anna."

"I'll place these things in the car, then. But what about the doctor? Have you heard from him?" "I called him, Corey. Now, I just have to wait until he returns my call. He has to sign the death certificate, before I call the undertaker. They require the signed certificate. 'There was NO NEED to call 9ll', as Michael would have said. No sense in trying to bring him back to life. I promised him--no resuscitation attempts. The doctors have both explained to me that his body functions were slowing down. Michael was prepared to die."

"He certainly didn't want all that fuss again. Can I stay with you? And Mike?"

"Oh, please do, Corey. That would mean a lot to me."

While Corey placed those few items in his car, I left a message on David's answering machine. I also notified Bob, as I had promised. I tried Lucy's number for one last time and gave up. Just at that moment, Beth, my friend from Calgary, phoned. She was in Toronto, waiting to be admitted for surgery. When I told her that Michael had just died, she offered to come to me. I was grateful for her support, but explained that Michael's body had not been removed. Beth provided her telephone number and gave me permission to call her at any time throughout that night. It didn't matter how late, she would come when I needed her.

CHAPTER FIVE

Although David did not call, Kim contacted me by nine o'clock. He explained that after Michael's remains had been taken, I was expected to meet them at Risha's to have dinner. The idea of food was a vague, distant concept to me. I refused their kind invitation--but Kim disregarded my objections. He insisted that he'd call me again, later.

Corey and I took turns being near Michael, or just standing in his bedroom doorway, observing his body in repose. We needed to stay close to him. Shortly after midnight, the doctor telephoned. His beeper had not been functioning during the evening. Within fifteen minutes, he arrived. Once I had escorted him into the apartment, he walked directly into Michael's bedroom.

"Oh, Mike, Mike. What a strange position you have yourself in, son. No matter. We'll leave you like that."

He ruffled Michael's brown, spikey hair with his hand, and patted his shoulder. Dr. Drake showed obvious affection and his eyes brimmed over with emotion. We looked at each other, he sighed and shook his head with sadness. I couldn't react, but remained rigidly still. As I looked at Michael's body, I saw that his body had altered in colour. There were red splotches of various sizes all along his body, close to the mattress, where his blood had pooled. A thin rivulet of blood leaked from his mouth and his skin had developed a grey, waxen, taut appearance. Could this used container--this shell--have held the lively, brilliant and loving entity that had been my Michael? Without his spirit, it was an empty husk, worn and discarded.

As the doctor walked towards me, I turned and stumbled into the dining room. My legs felt unsteady, as the final reality of Michael's loss overwhelmed everything else. I sunk into Michael's favourite chair at the table. Corey sat desolately on the black futon, by the window. He had been leafing through one of the art reference texts. Slowly, he raised his head and acknowledged Dr. Drake's presence with a nod and slight smile.

"This is Corey, Dr. Drake. He was Michael's friend."
"Yes, how are you doing?"
"Okay." Corey's voice caught in his throat, and he strangled a small cough.

I peered at Corey then and recognized the enormous impact of Mike's death upon him. His face was pale and drawn from strain. His dark eyes had an injured, guarded appearance. Corey's dejection and bereavement touched me deeply. We had both lost our dearest friend.

"Well, let's get this certificate filled out. It must be given to the attendants when they arrive. You realize that the major cause of death will be listed as dehydration, due to the vomiting and diarrhea?"

I nodded in affirmation, but couldn't respond. We were surely dreaming. At any moment, Michael would stagger out of the bedroom wearing his favourite green housecoat, to chide, "Knock it off. This has gone on long enough." Only a portion of me acknowledged his death. I would never again hear his voice, or see his smile. He would never turn and scowl, or put his head to one side and stare, when I did something foolish. How could Michael's life cease? Would mere memories suffice? The doctor's calm, resonant voice ripped me from my reverie.

"There were various complications of the disease which resulted in Michael's demise. I must stipulate that he was my patient during the past four to five years, and that he had full-blown AIDS."

"Can anyone have access to this knowledge?"
"It is privileged information."
"But statistics are compiled regarding the number of AIDS deaths in this city?"
"Yes. That is essential."
"Can 'Johnny Public' check on the actual cause of Mike's death? On the death certificate which will be released to me, will it state the cause of death as AIDS?"
"No, Maria. No, it will not. That document only contains a verification of the date and place of Michael's death. You'll use those when applying for death benefits, income tax purposes, insurance claims...that type of thing. This is a closed file, insofar as the AIDS disease is concerned. Your privacy, and Michael's, will be protected."
"Okay. You see, I'm still fighting like hell to ensure my privacy--Michael's privacy--Anna's right to discretion. Privacy won't always be so vital. Mike frequently claimed, 'Nobody cares, Ma. Nobody cares.' Maybe that's true, but I won't tolerate criticism of him. He was too special. David described Mike as, 'a complex and beautiful person'. Nobody can hurt him now. So many dead from AIDS. So many precious young people deteriorating, dying...not right. Not fair. Some day we'll heal, won't we Corey? No consolation...right now...grasp onto support...because...so much bigotry and hatred out there. This should teach love and understanding, instead. Let those ignorant asses witness such pain, such loneliness...excruciating...raw. Sorry, I'm rambling. I just can't..."

My voice broke. My thoughts whirled and rushed in discordant revolving circles. The quiet calm cacoon, in which I had contained myself since Michael's death, abruptly vanished into vertigo. Rationalization did not work. There was no need to be brave for Michael's sake. His vacant body remained in repose, teasing, as if he softly slept. Michael was dead.

That part of me that was invested in Michael, was also lost. Loving and caring for Michael had involved my strongest physical and emotional commitment. I had given Michael my time, my experience, my possessions, my strength and my love. Our bond was forged of vitality, sensitivity and intensity. Death had crushed that special familial and confidant relationship.

I had completed so much anticipatory grieving. Was I not prepared for this death? We had carefully reviewed all of the practical concerns. Together, we had planned to cushion these cruel aspects of his loss. Michael had accomplished loving farewells. I must permit him to go.

The doctor reached across the table and patted my arm, indicating sincere concern. Corey stood up and looked at me, uncertainly. He took a hesitent step forward and regarded me, beseechingly. Ashamed of my faltering reaction, I took a deep breath and forced myself to sit up straighter in the chair. I searched the doctor's eyes, and explained,

"I'm sorry. I'll be...just fine. I seem to go a little bit crazy every once in awhile." A nervous laugh escaped me.

"That's also normal. Sorrow causes many divergent reactions. Do you realize that you must call the funeral home now?"

I took a deep breath to prevent my serene mask from slipping. "Yes. I can take care of it."

"Please," Corey interjected, "Let me do that for you, Maria."

The doctor left hastily, and within twenty minutes the attendants rang the apartment buzzer. Corey ushered them into Michael's bedroom, and shut the door. While the two attendants were placing Michael within the black body bag, the little kitten that lived upstairs mewed and scratched at the dining room window. That grey and white ball of fur had visited Michael often, in the past two months. I had wiped away its muddy footprints from one end of the apartment to the other. I wondered if it sensed that Michael was dead.

They brought out Michael, tucked inside the black body bag, and tightly strapped to the wheeled cart by a secured belt. The bag seemed flattened, since Michael had been so frail and thin. IS THAT ALL THAT IS LEFT OF MY SON? I whimpered and promptly slipped away from the doorway. I didn't want to see it. I didn't want to watch them take my Michael away. The attendant moved steadily towards me.

"May I have the signed death certificate, left by the doctor, please?"

"Oh, yes...there...on the table." I remained rooted to the floor, unable to pass him the document.

"Thank you. Will you call the funeral home tomorrow, please, so that you will know the day and time of your son's cremation?"

I nodded, but could not speak.

Corey stood close beside me, observing us cautiously and staring at the body bag. He placed his hands upon his hips and made a strange, raspy gutteral sound. In a forced, brittle voice, he asked,

"What kind of car are you using for Mike?"
"It's a hearse."
"Yes, but what kind? Is it a Rolls?" His smile was tight and unnatural.

"As a matter of fact, it's a brand new one. It is a Rolls-Royce, and this is its first night to be used. Would you like to come out and see it?"

"Yes. Is it black?" He put his head to one side, and reminded me of Michael.

"That's right, sir. It's a fine vehicle. Won't you escort us out, and take a look?"

I slumped into the chair. As I did so, through the open door sauntered the little gray kitten from upstairs. It walked around and around the body bag on the cart three times, mewing pitifully. Corey stared at me, his brown eyes registering shock.

"Is that the kitten from upstairs that always visited Mike?"
"Often. I don't know its name. Michael just called it CAT. They were friends. He gave Mike comfort."
"It has come to say good-bye."
"Yes. Somehow it knows. Michael told me that CAT lowered his blood pressure and relaxed him. Stroking CAT soothed him, somehow. Go and check out the hearse, Corey. I'll stay here. Leave CAT. Maybe it wants to inspect the apartment."

The cat sprinted, leaped upon Michael's bed and sniffed at the spot where his body had been. It curled into a tight little ball for a brief moment, mewed raucously and scooted up the stairs after Corey. I shambled down the hall, groped up the stairs and leaned heavily against the door frame. The shining new hearse sat double-parked across the street. Michael lay inside it. After shaking the attendants' hands, Corey walked decisively towards me.

NOT A TOTAL WASTE

"Just like Mike, to go off in style." Corey gave me a lopsided, sad grin. "That was a brand new Rolls-Royce hearse!"
"Seems appropriate, doesn't it? Nothing but the best."

We smiled, as if to reinforce one another. Absently, I checked my watch. I was amazed to notice that it registered one o'clock in the morning. The telephone shrilled rudely, scathing our emotions in the vacant silence. Corey and I shuddered. Then, Kim's voice penetrated my thoughts,

"Well, sweetie, has the doctor arrived?"
"Yes, and the funeral home has just removed Michael. Corey has been with me all evening, taking care of details. I couldn't have coped without him. He leaving now, worn right out."
"Call a taxi, wear Michael's splendid new shirt with your blue jeans, and come over to Risha's. Your supper is waiting. Tell Corey that he is very welcome, too."
"I'm sorry, Kim." I covered my face with my hand, and brushed my hair away from my neck. "I couldn't eat anything. I'm very tired. Perhaps Corey would come."
"No, Maria, that won't do. No excuses at all. You must eat. Michael would want you to be with us. If you won't call a cab, we'll come and get you."
"No. Please. Don't do that. Oh...okay. I'll try. Corey is shaking his head, for no. He must rest."
"We're here--waiting for you. Hurry, now."

Somehow, I arrived at Risha's. Most of the staff were lounging on the patio chairs, chatting. The chef looked towards me, smiled as he gave me a 'thumb's up' gesture and said, "What do you know--the eagle has landed!" I looked beyond him, lowered my head, clenched my jaw and stubbornly shoved myself forward. How I yearned to sleep, without ever waking up again. An incredible isolation encircled me as I looked around the crowded patio at the laughing, jubilant people. Later, I must return to that empty apartment, and Michael would never be there, again. EMPTY. The apartment would forever be empty.

AFTERMATH

CHAPTER ONE

David and Kim huddled over their drinks, smoking Camel filtertips, at their favourite circular table in the front corner. This was the location always shared with Michael, reserved for them by the Maitre D'. At Mike's usual chair was arranged a place-setting of dishes and crystal wine goblets. David had requested that purposefully, for we must toast Mike on his spiritual journey. When I saw those provisions, the room tipped from one corner to the other and rapidly rotated. The limited walk from the door to the table suddenly expanded to become an extensive hike. HOLD ON. This excursion must be completed without a hitch. This, I owe Michael and his dear friends. Is this what grief is all about? BE SENSIBLE. DON'T BABBLE. BE CALM. FAKE IT.

David and Kim rose gallantly to greet me and I managed to seat myself. David's handsome, aristocratic features were pinched and strained. The overhead lights illuminated his fair hair and his hazel eyes shone with unshed tears. His countenance conveyed caring and concern. Kim appraised us cautiously from the sidelines, his features composed and reserved, providing strength and stability by his presence. I MUST NOT PERMIT THIS REPAST TO BECOME MELANCHOLY. David carried his own pain and Kim offered us empathy. I smiled faintly and nodded at them both.

"I could not call back, Maria. Thanks for your messages, but forgive my inability to respond. I'm sorry that I crumbled at the end."

"It's okay, David. You have been so helpful to both Michael and me. Kim explained that you were also grieving."

"Well, the kitchen has prepared something very special for you. Please try to eat. Have you had anything at all, today?"

"I honestly cannot remember. I think I had tea, once. Just had no appetite. Food was simply the last thing..."

"Corey stayed with you all evening?"

I turned to Kim to answer his query. My vision seemed so very clear one moment, and fuzzy the next. It was as if I had taken a drug with codeine, and it was causing an allergic reaction.

"Ummm. Well, Corey called about 6:30, I think. Michael died at 6:10. Then, Corey arrived close to 7 o'clock. I'm not sure. He kept me company...held me up, I suppose. We didn't expect it to take the entire evening. I'm sorry that I've kept you waiting all this time."

"Don't give it a thought. David arranged things with the manager."

Suddenly, it dawned on me that this restaurant was not supposed to be open at this late hour. Instantly, the waiter brought me the most amazing chicken broth that I had ever tasted. It was so thick and rich that my spoon had to be shoved through it. A platter of fine cheeses, fresh fruits, and my favourite vice--thick slabs of chocolate brownies, dripping with rich frosting, was placed in the centre of the table. It must have been extravagantly expensive for David to provide for this catering at such a late hour. This was a tribute to Michael. This was a unique wake. David's social astuteness and generosity were beyond my comprehension. Michael knew that I felt like "Alice in Wonderland", whenever I was fortunate to be part of their dining assemblage. Here I sat, a country bumpkin from the far northwest, wearing Michael's special shirt, sitting in one of Toronto's top restaurants at a peculiar hour in the morning, and celebrating the loss of my only son. Feeling beyond bewildered, I searched deeply into their faces. I saw their shared pain, and then my tears started in earnest.

Despite any discomfort at my overt display, they spoke gently as they guided food towards me. One by one, their strong hands reached forward to place succulent morsels into my mouth. Stunned and stupid, I opened my mouth to accept their offerings. Their supportive love encompassed me, and gradually the sharp, vise-like constriction that had been squeezing my throat and chest dissipated.

This despair was not mine alone. David and Kim reached out to me, surrounded my hands with their larger ones, and patiently waited for me to grasp a corner of my sanity and persist. I cannot recall much more of that dinner. The compassion and acceptance of David and Kim, the array of fine foods and rare wines have become a vague dream. Locked in my mind, however, are some of David's comments.

"You must not regress, Maria. You owe it to Michael's memory to find new hope, new meaning and purpose in his death. He would want you to harness this experience, value it and put it to some good use."

I only stared back. What possible good could result from his death? How could I fill a void? There was only black nothingness, now. I wanted to reply with Michael's stock phrase, THERE IS NO NEED. NOT ANY MORE. THERE IS NO NEED.

"Are you listening to David, Maria? Do you hear what he is trying to say?"

I gaped back at Kim, inanely.

"You have the grandchildren to think about. Michael adored those two kids. He thought of them constantly, and spoke of them with great admiration. Their future has to be planned and considered, now. You can't give up. Do you hear me? You have to turn things around, now. You have to put your sorrow to work in a positive manner. It cannot engulf you."

"David--wait--they'll be fine. They have their parents. They didn't get to be such great kids, on their own. None of them need me. Anna has her own life to lead. Bruce will not miss me. You expect me to make this grief work. Well, I can't. I don't have the guts. My motivation has shrivelled. I'm not so tough, after all. When my parents died, it hurt. When I lost three little babies, one after the other, the pain was raw. But, David that pain was a pittance, compared to Michael's death. To lose him, while he still had so much to live for...when he had so many talents to share with the world...so much love to offer..."

"Michael would have wanted you to deal constructively with his death. He was proud of you. Remember the many things that he taught you. Don't let go. Maria, don't besmirch his memory."

I froze. I stared at them vacantly. They knew. I did not want to go on, without Michael. Why was I alive and healthy, when he was dead? He was a far better person than I could ever become. If only I had fed him better, or been able to visit him more frequently so that he would not have been lonely. If only I had insisted that he have better home care. If only...I could execute a personal, quick exit. I moistened my lips with my tongue, and tried to mollify David.

"Don't worry. I'll be fine."

"You could study French. Michael always wanted you to pick that up again. You could go to Paris, and take a course where he had studied."

"Ummhmm."

"You could find a positive way to invest your experience with Michael's AIDS death, to help others. Take your energies and rechannel them, to encourage others who are grieving. You know that this plague is not over yet. We're only seeing the tip of the iceberg. Think of the many mothers who will lose their children because of AIDS. Michael yearned to prevent the destruction of families which he feared would become a catastrophic result. You could be instrumental in assisting others who must still struggle through the death of their loved one. Michael said that you were a real survivor. Prove that he was right."

I wanted to leap onto the table and shout, STOP. How could I plan ahead? Michael had needed my help...but he contributed more than his share, in return. He valued life. No one but Michael ever asked, "How are you doing? How are you feeling? Want to talk about it?" He'd never be there, for me, again. Nor for any of his friends. This intense loss was too private, too personal, too overwhelming, to be beneficial to strangers. Society's demands would be an added burden, too heavy for me to lift.

I recall toasting Michael with rare French wine. Or did I only dream of that? I clearly remember the kindness and empathy shown by David and Kim. Somehow, I returned to the apartment. Michael's soiled bed sheets, bloodied by the drippings from his mouth and the manipulations required to place his body within that black zippered bag, were stripped away. Automatically, I remade his bed. In a daze, I wandered through the apartment, caressed his possessions, and imagined him everywhere.

After three o'clock, I heard the phone ringing down the hall. Beth and Terry came to me, then. We sat at the dining room table until six the following morning, talking and weeping together. They offered intensive listening. They neither judged me, nor advised me. With open arms and hearts filled with love, they drank my putrid coffee and supported my suffering. When the sun rose, they left.

CHAPTER TWO

I lay on Michael's bed, in the spot where his body had been. His green duvet was wrapped snugly around me. I watched the sun make bizarre shapes on the ceiling, as he must have done before me. I scanned his bookshelves. Michael had been a talented, complex man. His art works were near the top, and those took some time to study in detail. So many abilities, encompassed within one individual. So much living, completed within a brief span.

The phone rang again, and this time it was Paul phoning, from Kelowna. Beth had called him and expressed concern for my well-being. I felt a bit defensive, initially, as though I should not convey the real turmoil my emotions were undergoing. But Paul was a friend, a wished-for big brother. He would serve as my non-evaluative audience, without expecting perfection. He knew my flaws, and could still tolerate me. We must have talked for an hour. No, I babbled and sobbed, without shame. Paul cajoled...listened... comforted. I emptied my soul.

Around ten o'clock that morning, Corey returned with Ted. They had brought packing boxes and assisted with the enormous job of sorting Michael's belongings. Throughout the humid heat of that day, without complaint, they persisted with the packing tasks. Anna called and promised to come the next morning. She was dealing with Michael's loss, too, in her own way. Ryan came downstairs and offered his help, as well. Somehow, the work would be completed. As we sorted items, Michael's friends selected special momentos among his possessions. Ted had particularly wanted the black leather jacket, which Michael had bought in Italy. Each person seemed to wish specific items, which held unique memories and comfort for them alone. It gave me pleasure to know that his possessions were not abandoned, but would be cherished by his friends and loved ones.

I had written Michael's obituary beforehand, and Bruce delivered it to the newspaper at home. He had also notified the school that I would be absent. Francine called Monday night to share my anguish at Michael's loss. I missed Bruce. I needed him.

Tuesday morning the funeral home notified me that Michael's cremation would be completed at 11:45 that morning. I declined attending. Previously, I had waived any necessity for verifying the corpse before the actual ceremony. First I called Anna, then Bruce, and then Bruce's mother. Until the cremation was completed, I sat silently in solitude, mentally bargaining with God. I begged for forgiveness, love and protection. A strange sensation of isolation engulfed me, as if I sat alone in a sound proof space capsule. No distracting sounds penetrated my thoughts. The world paused until Michael's bones were burned to dust.

I forced myself to continue packing for the rest of that day, vigorously filling boxes that had been left by Ted and Corey. I felt haggard and dishevelled by eleven that night, and thought I might actually sleep. Since Michael's death, I had merely cat-napped and eaten sparingly. My appearance was bedraggled. After rehanging Michael's good shirt, I noticed that I had been wearing the same rumpled jeans and one soiled matching blouse. It shocked me to realize that I had neither changed that blouse, nor bathed since Michael's death. My appearance was usually tidy; this relapse was amazing. I had even dozed wearing this outfit. I collapsed on Michael's bed, wrapped myself again in his duvet and hoped that I would finally fall into a deep sleep. I wanted sleep to erase all pain, and eradicate reality.

The phone rang repeatedly, supportive loving calls from caring friends who had heard the news about Michael. Francine called back and wanted to know what incomplete tasks she could undertake. An editorial filler from the New York Times was so reflective of Michael's own values, that I wanted to share it. Francine consented to read it at the memorial service. It was entitled, What we Learn from Illness, and went as follows:

"The ultimate value of illness is that it teaches us the value of being alive; this is why the ill are not just charity cases, but a presence to be valued. Illness and, ultimately, death remind us of living. 'The way we look to a distant constellation/That's dying in a corner of the sky,' Paul Simon sang. We look like a flicker of light. In the moment of that light going out, we learn that what counts is to keep it burning. Death is no enemy of life; it restores our sense of the value of living. Illness restores the sense of proportion that is lost when we take life for granted. To learn about value and proportion we need to honor illness, and ultimately to honor death."

After chatting with Francine, I cosied down into the bed clothes, closed my eyes, and finally slept. Around three o'clock in the morning I was awakened by the sound of a key in the front door lock. It was tried twice; then, the keys were dropped. An angry expletive was uttered, the keys were rattled, and one more effort was made to enter the apartment. I sat in silent terror in Michael's corner of the bed and waited, shivering. Only his friends possessed keys. On the day of his death, I had followed Bruce's request and changed the locks. He did not want me to remain in the apartment alone, otherwise. The meaningless epithet which I had overheard, had been from a feminine-sounding voice. I had no idea who stood outside, but I was afraid. What did they want? If they were friends, why had they not called? If they desired a momento to remind them of Michael, they only had to ask. Maybe it was an apartment dweller, tipsy from partying, who had tried this door in error. I tried to dismiss my irrational fear, and remain calm. However, I huddled in the corner, hugging my knees, enwrapped in Michael's duvet and trembled.

They did not knock, or try to enter the back door. They left. Despite the late hour, I phoned Anna. She was not asleep. She and Bernie had a guest. They were sharing Michael's unfinished bottle of whiskey which we had located underneath the kitchen sink, and chatting. I was not the only one having difficulty sleeping. When I detailed the key episode, Bernie insisted on coming to get me immediately. I promptly acquiesced. Before I realized it, I was asleep next to Jenni. At six o'clock the next morning I returned to the city by taxi. Ted arrived by eight o'clock to continue helping me with the packing.

On Wednesday Anna, Bernie and the children arrived, around ten o'clock. Bernie had been returning most days to remove filled boxes. Anna had the additional task of trying to determine the right spot for everything, once Bernie got the truck unloaded. It must have been painful for her to go through all of that rigmorole of packing and unpacking her only brother's belongings. That morning, Jenni and Sean volunteered to escort me to the funeral home to fetch Michael's urn. I fought hard to provide the appearance of normalcy, for this task. Once we got there, they looked about the large waiting room, with genuine interest.

"I like this place, where you brought Uncle Mike, Nana. They sure do have nice furniture."

"Nana, look at the pretty rug. It has every colour. Did you notice the big dish with all the candies?"

"Can we have some, Nana?"

"Yes, you may help yourselves. That's why they leave them there--for grandchildren to select their favourites."

"Do lots of grandchildren come here, Nana?"

"Not lots. But some."

"How many can we have?"

"I think you should do as Uncle Michael used to, when he was a little boy. You should pick one for each hand, and one for your pocket."

"Nana, where did they put Uncle Mike?"

The director walked in at that moment with some forms for me to sign, and carried Michael's urn. When I attempted to pick up the urn, I realized its surprising weight.

"Nana, is Uncle Mike in there?"

"Yes, Jenni. He is."

"Is that shiny box heavy?"

"Very heavy, Sean."

"What's it made of, Nana?"

"It is brass. That's a kind of metal."

Sean clicked his fingers, said, "Oh, Boy!" Then they both moved around me and the urn encompassed within my arms, in a circle. They giggled happily, and to my amazement, Sean said, "Just like Uncle Mike! He did like his HEAVY METAL music." For a moment I was completely baffled, and then dissolved into laughter. The director watched with a puzzled air, shrugged and left the room. I knew that I had to get the children out of there, before I ended up in nervous hysteria. Clutching the death certificates and the urn close to my body, we headed down the front steps. At the bottom, Sean said,

"Look over there, Nana. A restaurant."
"Yes. What about it, dear?"
"Nana, we're starving. Can we please have some lunch?"
"Oh, honey, of course! You both hold onto my arms, and we'll get across the traffic."
"Jenni, you hold onto Nana's arm. I'm going to stop those damn cars."

Before I could call him back, Sean held up his arms and made the cars stop. I felt as though, at any moment, they would start rolling again. We followed Sean safely, like Moses' people, with traffic parted on either side of us--at a standstill. The entire experience had seemed to occur at a great distance. I felt stunned, and divorced from reality. Once we were seated at a booth in the restaurant, Sean said,

"Nana, please place Uncle Mike on the seat beside you. Then, when the waitress comes, she won't get spooked about him being with us."
"Oh. I guess it could put somebody off, a bit."
"You just rest, Nana. I'll do the ordering."
"Do you know what you want, Jenni? Tell Sean."
"I'm just hungry, Sean. I don't want any of that cabbage cut up stuff, okay?"
"You mean cole slaw. No problem."

The young waitress walked up to the booth with her pencil and pad, prepared to take our orders. She stood and looked at me, and smiled. I made a futile effort to respond. Sean efficiently took over.

"I'll do the ordering please, lady. We'll have three toasted westerns on brown. No cole slaw. Just milk for me and for Jenni. And please bring Nana coffee. She just loves her coffee."

The waitress and I shared a smile, and I nodded. She said, "Thank you, sir."
Sean turned to Jenni, and said,
"See how easy that was?"
Jenni looked at him, frowned and faced me.
"Can I order next time, Nana? Girls can order, too."
"Certainly, dear."
"You can pay, too, Jenni. Equal rights."
"Now, Sean, don't tease. Here comes your food."

They ate with zest. I sipped my coffee, but felt no appetite for the sandwich.

"Nana, are you saving that sandwich for Uncle Mike?"
"No, Sean, I'm just not hungry. Do you think that you and Jenni could share it?"
"Sure we could."

The waitress came over to refill my cup, and Sean said,
"I would like to order again, please, lady. We'll have three more of those good westerns, but no more milk."
"Oh, kids, I'm sorry," I interjected. "I didn't realize that you were so hungry. What else would you like, besides westerns?"
"Nana, get real. These aren't for me and Jenni. These are to take with us, for my Mom and Dad. My Mom is a basket case. She's not cooking, lately. They're sure hungry, too, Nana."
I nodded at the waitress, and said, "To go, please."

When it was time to leave, Sean said,
"You ladies just stay inside the door where it's cooler. I'll stop a taxi for us. Let's go."
"I have to go to the toilet, Sean."
"I should have known, Jenni. I think you plan it that way. Now you watch, Nana, there'll be four taxis go past while she's in the bathroom, and then we'll never find another one."

NOT A TOTAL WASTE

I laughed at such cynicism from a ten-year-old young man, but it took at least ten minutes for another taxi to appear. Sean decided that he would nuke the sandwiches in the microwave for his parents' lunches. It felt as though we were situated within the eye of a hurricane. Normal daily events unfolded, despite the whirling chaos which surrounded us.

CHAPTER THREE

That night, I had dinner with David and Kim. David surprised me with an exquisite pair of blue sapphire, gold-set stud earings from Birks. These were a gift from him and Michael. He gave me a photo of Michael which I had not seen before, and a copy of the POEMS OF PAUL CELAN, Translated from the German. One poem had been selected by David for an obituary. It read as follows:

"THREAD SUNS
above the grey-black wilderness.
A tree-
high thought
tunes in to light's pitch: there are
still songs to be sung on the other side
of mankind."

We shared a lovely dinner and a supportive, relaxing visit. I knew that I would miss these precious friends of Michael, very much. They were more than links to Michael; they had become my friends, too.

Thursday developed into a final, hard push to get the end of the packing and moving accomplished. I worked steadily throughout the day and Bernie removed the filled boxes. Anna continued with her double job of emptying one apartment, and relocating those items within her townhouse. Enough empty boxes remained for me to expect completion of the packing by the following morning.

Around four o'clock, Ryan came downstairs to tell me that Lynda had returned from Thunder Bay and was taking Michael's death hard. I invited them to share dinner, as my guests, that evening. Corey and Ted appeared and offered to assist with last minute packing. How weary and wan they seemed, from the stress of Michael's death and all of the help which they had given to me. They agreed to share the dinner party, too. Corey reserved a table for us at a restaurant on Parliament Street, which he and Michael had often frequented. Ryan explained that he had called another friend of Michael's, Allan, and had invited him to come along. We were delighted as the numbers grew. Allan had studied in Rome with Michael, Ryan and Lynda. This was shaping up to become a spontaneous and enjoyable party.

Although initially unplanned, this "wake" became a joyful celebration. For the first time since Michael's death, I laughed until my jaws ached. The funny experiences which were related, regarding their studies in Europe and in Toronto, offered unique insights into many of the good times which Michael had enjoyed before his illness. It was uplifting to know that he'd done so many interesting things and had so much fun. Their merry adventures helped to erase my concerns related to Michael's isolation and loneliness during the last two years of his life. Michael had actually packed in so many exhilarating experiences, in such a short life span. Obviously, he had also made some fine, lasting friendships.

Friday morning, I left the apartment by nine o'clock. I took the photograph, which David had given to me, to a photography studio on Spadina. Copies were made for the church altar and for Michael's friends. While these were being prepared, I used that interim to have the lenses changed in Michael's "John Lennon" spectacles, to my own prescription. It had been a re-cycling suggestion made by Michael. The lighter frames would eliminate head-aches after a heavy day of marking students' work.

These duties were completed shortly before noon and I returned to the apartment. My few belongings and Michael's art work were packed. Michael's urn was placed in a worn piece of his luggage. With Bernie's next load, the apartment would be vacant. The rooms echoed in a dismal, distressing manner.

I took one last sojourn around the apartment and peeked through the white-enamelled security bars of the front room window. This had been my vantage point as I had awaited Michael's return from his last bike ride, when he had fallen down the stairs. Across the street had sat the Rolls Royce hearse which had removed Michael's body bag. From the kitchen window, I peered onto the patio and recalled the raccoons and a myriad of other events. I scanned the familiar kitchen and caressed the glossy counter tops which Michael had built. The apartment held many potent memories, yet it appeared hollow and forlorn, now. With regret, I unplugged Michael's telephone from the bedroom socket and placed it inside my handbag. Purposefully, I reached for the two small suitcases and balanced their weight carefully.

After closing the door softly behind me for the last time, I headed towards the end of Berkley Street. I refrained from looking back, but pushed solidly forward. The tall spreading chestnut trees which Michael had loved sheltered the street, forming a canopy which nearly met in the centre. On the same corner where Michael and I had frequently waited, I hailed a taxi and headed for the airport. Michael's urn was safely stowed within the bag, on the seat beside me. Preparations for his memorial service awaited confirmation. It was time, now, to take my Michael home.

CHAPTER FOUR

Bruce met my plane, and carried my luggage to the car. We spoke little on the drive back home, but he patted my knee in a comforting gesture.

"I'm sorry that I couldn't be there to help. I just couldn't handle it."

"Umhmm."

"Do you still plan to have a memorial service here? Is it really necessary?"

"Yes. I have it pretty well arranged, already. Francine helped me."

"Do I have to be there?"

"I want you to be there. I expect you to be with me. Frankly...because...oh, it's up to you. This service if for us and for Michael. He deserves a proper farewell. I hope that the closure will hasten our healing process. Also, Michael's friends should have a chance to say good-bye".

"Most of them have left town to find jobs, or to complete their education. Why you need to go to all of this fuss, when you are so tired, makes no sense..."

"You don't get it, do you? I know that there are still people who care for Michael, in this city. They have asked about him, during the past two years. We also have friends, acquaintances and students, who want an opportunity to show that they are sorry. People are saddened at Michael's death and wish to express that to us. It's no secret that we are hurting like hell. We could sure use the sympathy and support which they will offer. It's about love, Bruce, and a sharing of our pain. There's more compassion out there, than you realize."

"It seems like a lot of unnecessary work. You can't bring him back. He's dead."

"Michael deserves a loving, respectful send-off. His bravery was formidable. I have never met anyone so gutsy..." My voice broke, and I blinked back angry tears.

"Okay. Let it go. If you want to do this, then its all right by me. I don't see what purpose all of this serves, but I'll go along with your plans. I'd rather not attend, that's all."

How could I explain the value of friendship, at this time? We were both reeling from the hurt of losing Michael. The support and caring of friends would ease our anguish. Bruce's apparent withdrawal from the reality of Michael's illness and death, could not erase the event. Michael's death was a high wall of throbbing pain that we must somehow pass through. Once on the other side, maybe we could pick up the pieces of our lives, and go on. Perhaps not.

In an effort to block out Bruce's response, I concentrated on the beautiful scenery as we drove homeward. The trees on the distant hills were freshly green, as only early June can paint them. This was the colour of the green wool which Michael had selected for his hand-knitted cardigan that I made for him when he started kindergarten. This was Michael's favourite colour and season of the year. The myriad verdant shadings showed tender, delicate hues, which made the forest seem almost translucent. Cadmium lemon yellow, mixed with cerulean blue, were blended beautifully. The effects of the sunlight on the forest touched those shades of springtime and their bursting buds. Additional deciduous trees, further along in their development, gloried in their seasonal transformation.

High branches, already spread widely under lush foliage of a darker, richer green, glowed as they filtered out the sunlight. Light and dark Hookers green, shaded with brown, mellowed those richer values. Pine and spruce trees stretched eagerly towards the sunlight, appearing as indistinct, softly-blurred outlines. Only a subtle change was obvious in their colours throughout this season, but the larches wore their bright foliage proudly. The little streams along the side of the highway bubbled merrily, still high from the melting

NOT A TOTAL WASTE

bush snows. June was a fresh, beautiful month in Northwestern Ontario. The delightful smell of freshly-cut grass drifted through the slightly open window. Bedding plants in front gardens were beginning to show blossoms, which nodded their heads in the intermittent breeze. This was a truly delightful day in which to bring Michael home.

After unpacking, I sorted through a fistful of accumulated telephone messages. One from the priest required an immediate response. The memorial service was scheduled for Tuesday, at four o'clock in the afternoon. When I contacted the priest, he agreed to come to the house the next afternoon to discuss the final arrangements.

The next day, Bruce joined us in the front room to assist with those preparations.

"The service will include the Holy Eucharist, of course?"
"No. We won't have communion."
"Why not? Was this a suicide?"
"We do not want the consecrated bread and wine used, since many of our friends are not of this faith. They would be uncomfortable. Let's avoid any additional awkwardness. Frankly, Father, I have never felt personally secure about numerous people imbibing from the same cup."
"Pardon me?"
"It's just my own personal reflection on the single cup, being passed from one to another. I've felt this discomfort ever since I accepted the communion cup from a woman who was terminally ill with cancer. I've also read about the spread of tuberculosis among our native people over the years, and wondered how large a role the communion cup has played. I see so much mononucleosis among my students, and hepatitis is prevalent. I don't believe that wine is potent enough to destroy viral infections, and don't wish to pass on any illness. Tuberculosis and cancer are considered to be viruses-- and there are lots of other diseases which we don't fully understand. I just refuse to place anyone in jeopardy. I can't accept responsibility for a disease transference at Michael's memorial service."
"I'm amazed that you feel that way. Such a response is highly unusual. I have never heard of such a..."
"It's a personal thing. Complex, maybe...but...HUMOUR ME!"

The priest stared at me, and then turned his gaze upon Bruce. He said nothing initially, and then asked with a trace of irritation,

"Do you feel the same way, Bruce? After all..."
"It's up to Maria."
"I see. Well, I thought that we would perhaps offer the following hymn..."
"If you don't mind, I prefer the hymn which stipulates that Michael's limbs and hands are expected to be whole again...that he is truly without pain...and that he has consecrated himself, his body, his soul, his intellect, to God. I don't know the name of the hymn. I remember that it goes something like..."
"Oh, of course, I know that piece, well. You needn't try to sing it. Of course, if that is the one which you wish to select, it's no problem. It is hardly one used for funerals, or memorial services, but if it is what you wish..."
"Yes, and did Francine contact you, Father? You are aware that three friends have offered to sing? The organist is familiar with the music, apparently. 'Amazing Grace', 'Clouds', and 'When You Walk Through a Storm', are the renditions which they have prepared. Did Francine clarify that she would complete a reading? Will you also have a lay reader?"
"Well, look, let's respond to each question, one by one, here. Yes, Francine has contacted me, and all arrangements have been taken care of, relating to the music. Two of those pieces are actually more secular than ecumenical, you understand. That seems to be your choice, Maria. What about this reading from Francine? What is its subject matter? Is it ecclesiastical, or worldly?"
"The hymn, the songs, and the readings have been selected because they are representative of particular stages in Michael's lifetime. The Psalm which I have chosen is the twenty-third, by the way. These are appropriate, if you had known our son, Father".
"I see. The reading? You haven't explained its source."
"That has come from a book written by Arthur Frank, while he battled cancer. It was quoted in the New York Times, just a week before Michael's death."
"And it relates to? What?"
"It is extremely representative of Michael's values, and his courage. It discusses the pertinence of appreciating our health, honouring illness, and respecting death. Michael felt that death should remind us to esteem life. He was not afraid to die."
"I see. Are you in agreement, Bruce? Are you comfortable with these preparations?"

NOT A TOTAL WASTE

I regarded them both with amazement. I was not requesting permission. These plans were determined, as far as I was concerned. This meeting was merely for confirmation, not for discussion or negation. Bruce regarded me cautiously, and my incredulity must have been apparent. Bruce flushed, cleared his throat, and quickly left the room. He wanted no part of this deliberation.

"You know, there are other Psalms, as well as the twenty-third, which you might prefer. Some consider it to be hackneyed, by indiscriminate use. For example, there is the..."

"Please...I'm not interested. Michael loved the twenty-third Psalm, because of its comforting familiarity. It may seem trite to some, but not to him. Nor to me. I also would like you to read from a book of poetry, which I had located among Michael's books. You could select whichever poem you deem to be appropriate, from this Gibran text."

"Oh. This is not commonly done, but I can certainly go through the book and select one which should suffice."

"Thank you. I did indicate some of Michael's preferences, but you should cull the one which you think is best."

"It's my pleasure. Is there anything else, then?"

"Yes. This poem was selected by Michael's friend, and translated from the German. It is to go on the front cover of the liturgy folder, with this photograph of Michael below it. I will place additional mailing copies, printed on heavy bond, in the narthex. Someone may wish them as momentos."

"That's unusual. We ordinarily place the church's photograph on the front of that document. Besides, it is costly to have those printed."

"Fine. I will readily cover that. I understand that my sorority sisters have generously offered to prepare a post-service luncheon, in the church basement?"

"Oh yes, that's been arranged. The lay reader will be available, as well. "

"I would like to write cheques now, for the lay reader, the printing costs, the organist, and for you. Are there any other costs, which I may have overlooked?"

"Well, no. You seem to have given careful thought to most of those plans. May I ask just what caused your son's death?"

"Michael died of AIDS, Father. When people ask, we say that he died of cancer. That is not an untruth, since he had cancer scattered throughout his body. He'd also had a stroke, and was partially paralyzed. His heart stopped. Michael went to sleep, quietly, beside me. Why? Are you homophobic? Does it upset you, giving a service for an AIDS-related death?"

"Oh. Of course not. You have not made public his AIDS problem?"

"It wasn't a problem. It was a disease, which killed Michael. It's not necessary to discuss this, nor to pass judgment."

"Was Michael homosexual?"

"His sexual preference is no-one else's business. WE HAVE LOST OUR ONLY SON, FATHER. MICHAEL HAS DIED A HORRIBLE DEATH. The name of the disease is of small importance. He suffered a long, lingering and cruel death, and showed himself to be strong and courageous. His loss, and our grief are what we are contending with here."

"Of course."

"Michael deserves the best service possible. He was the most uncomplaining, resilient human being that I have ever known. Michael was also our child. He was only thirty-three--still such a young man. He will always be my baby. OUR ONLY SON." The tears flowed, unchecked down my face.

"Uh, well, yes, I see. Do you have any particular ideas as to where or how you wanted Michael's urn to be placed?"

"Yes, Father. I would like the urn to be placed on the altar railing, at the centre, as close to the altar as possible."

"It is unethical for it to be placed upon the altar."

"Fine. This large, framed photograph of Michael should be placed, with a few flowers, to one side of the urn, also close to the altar--perhaps on a small table. On the opposite side, I wish to place a framed Botticelli tapestry. Michael brought the artwork home from Florence, Italy for me and I spent two years completing the needlepoint work. He loved the Italian architecture, art, countryside and people. If he had lived, he would have retired there. I've had the tapestry placed in a gilded, Baroque-style frame and I will order an engraved plaque. I wish this needlepoint to be dedicated in Michael's memory and given to the church."

"A tapestry? Where is this? May I see it?"

I escorted the priest down the hall towards our master bedroom, to show him the completed Mother and Child tapestry which hung over my desk. He walked up to it, nodded in approval and removed the heavy picture from the wall. He carried it in his arms, down the hall to the front room.

"Yes. It will do nicely. Very nicely."

NOT A TOTAL WASTE
_____235

"I'm so glad. I was uncertain whether you would approve of the Madonna and Child theme. However, since you have frequently stressed the family church elements, it seemed appropriate. Michael selected this tapestry while he studied architecture in Rome and Florence. I feel contented to part with it, as a memorial tribute to Michael."

"This is truly beautiful work. I think that...well, I am sure that we can find someplace for it. Perhaps in the narthex of the church. I don't know too much about art. Now, please call me if there's anything else that you might want to discuss. If you are concerned about anything at all, contact me directly. I assume that you have ordered flowers for the altar?"

"Yes, Father. Red roses and stephanotis. Two vases, for either side of the altar."

"Fine. Call me if you need me. Otherwise, I guess I will see you, close to four o'clock, on Tuesday."

"I will initially arrive shortly after three o'clock, Father, to ensure that everything is in place and to bring Michael's urn."

"Oh, yes, of course. Where is Bruce? I'd like to say good-bye and express my sympathy to him."

"He's in the bathroom. You'll see him Tuesday, perhaps."

"Oh...oh...Fine. Call me, should you need me."

"Thanks, Father."

I closed the door softly, went back into the front room and collapsed in an easy chair. Trying to settle all of those tiny, piquant details had drained me. I experienced relief that things had been set in motion, and that preparations were confirmed. Nevertheless, I wished that Bruce had remained beside me. I had wanted his affirmation while I clarified my concepts to the Priest. I was uncertain whether my ideas were acceptable, as viewed by the church. I had instinctively determined what had been correct for Michael's tribute. It would be a beautiful, uplifting service, which would remind those present that we cannot take our loved ones or our lives for granted...that we must value our loved ones, while we have them...and that the terminally ill deserve our respect, empathy and love. The service would convey that impact. Our friends would offer their needed support and affection.

I heard Bruce come slowly down the hallway. I kept my eyes closed and my head rested against the back of the chair. I was deeply exhausted.

"He's gone, then? Did you get it settled, the way that you wanted?"

"Yes, but you sure weren't much help. He's YOUR priest. It's YOUR church. Surely to God, you could have helped me." In frustration, I scolded him.

"I don't understand what you want. Don't be irritated with me. I was just in the way. How could I have helped?"

"By just bloody-well being in the room, instead of running off down the hall."

"You don't have to get nasty. This has nothing to do with me. I see no point in any of it."

"Really? It must be nice to be able to separate yourself from the whole damned world and isolate yourself from familial obligations."

"That's not fair. I've done what I could."

"That's not good enough. I needed your support--emotionally, and physically. So did Michael. I disliked having to assert my requests for his memorial service. I have never felt comfortable, even though I changed my religious affiliations over thirty years ago. You know that I've tried. It is so important that this service be right, for Michael. It just can't be messed up. This is a service for the living, as well as the dead. Can't you understand that?"

He stood staring at me, with a pale, still face. His blue-grey eyes held unshed tears, and his lack of any outward emotion frightened me. He would grieve in his own manner, in his own time, and I had no right to push him into this sensitive catharsis. I felt sorry that he could not emote readily, to relieve some of the pain which he must be experiencing. I watched him steadily and waited for a response. How I yearned for him to cross the chasm between us and hold me in his arms. I wished for his reassurance that some day everything would be all right again and that we would survive this trauma together. Calmly, he crossed his arms in front of his chest and rocked his incisors against his lower teeth. He seemed to be assessing me and finding me lacking. Rejection seemed to be the opposite of love. Without any sufficient reason, I snapped. I simply lost it. I tasted the bile of hot anger in my mouth, jumped up and rushed towards him.

"Damn you. DAMN YOU. You're just never there, when I need you. Don't stand still, glaring at me! How dare you. How could you leave me to tend Michael all that time, without any help?

Where were you while I dealt with his death, his cremation, his packing, and now all of his service arrangements. You're never there, when I need you. Never."

I struck him. I had not previously raised my hand to him. Now, I used both of my hands, made into tight fists and I pummelled his chest, over and over again. He accepted the repeated pounding. He neither flinched, nor moved. No effort was made to protect himself. I flailed at him until I had no strength left to punch him again. Horror swept over me as I became aware of my actions. I sunk to my knees before him, covered my face with my hands and wept bitterly. I moaned and rocked myself, trying to provide some solace, while I dealt with the shame of my violence. In all of our years of marriage, I had never raised my hand to him, or to our children. Why now? This brutal punishment afflicted us both. How could he tolerate this abuse, without any sign of emotion?

He pivoted, moved away and headed back down the hall. He remained there, until I had stopped weeping. I sat sniffling and hiccuping in the chair, when he returned. I could not look into his face, or speak. Physical battering had never been a part of our lives. He did not utter a word, but stood quietly in front of me, evaluating me.

"Oh, God, Bruce. What's happened to us? How could you stand for me to act in that manner? I am so sorry. So ashamed. I don't know what to say."
"Well, that's a change. Do you feel any better?"
"I feel terrible. Ugly. Mean. And sorry. I'm very sorry."
"I forgive you."

Without looking at him, I fled past him to the bedroom. Emotionally spent, I fell across my bed and cried myself to sleep. He had readily forgiven me, yet my heart would not relinquish my pain. I grasped onto my anger tightly, unable to yield.

I recall little about that Sunday. We existed. On Monday morning, I returned to school to supervise examinations and to pick up my students' papers. As if in a trance, I marked exams and calculated final marks throughout that night. Early Tuesday morning, I submitted my marks to the Guidance Department. By one o'clock I excused myself to prepare for Michael's memorial service.

On the way home, I had purchased an exquisite hand-made floral wreath. It was made of dried flowers, in predominant soft hues of blue and green and was hung immediately on the front door. When I was a child, a house of mourning would have been decorated with a large black ribbon across the doorway and a massive, dark wreath. I decided that this mass of flowers was a joyful statement on Michael's life. After collecting Michael's urn, and his large framed photograph, Bruce and I drove to the church to reassure ourselves that everything was ready.

The priest was completing the liturgy folders. The organist carefully ran through the music, and luncheon was being placed attractively upon the downstairs tables. The lay reader, attired in his long white surplice, was engrossed in his reading material. After murmured greetings, we departed unobstrusively.

After showering, I stood before my closet and tried to determine what I should wear. The black crepe shift, with the white satin trim, was discarded because its effect was too morbid. Instead, I selected a creamy off-white linen suit, black silk blouse, white hose and off-white leather pumps. White was the funeral colour of the Japanese, and on this humid, hot day it seemed to be a sensible choice. I wore the sapphire stud earings which David and Michael had given to me and a small sapphire pendant. The creamy-white pillbox hat was vetoed. Instead, my hair was brushed and sprayed lightly, against the high humidity.

Bruce showered and dressed in grey flannels, blue blazer, white shirt and a silver/blue-striped University of Toronto tie. This was similar to the outfit which he had worn to our marriage, the children's baptisms, their graduations and Anna's wedding. It seemed fitting that he would wear it on this important occasion, too.

We spoke not at all during our drive to the church, as both of us were lost in our own remembrances. When Bruce reached over and patted my knee in a reassuring motion, I was too numb to respond.

CHAPTER FIVE

The service was perfect. Each single step followed smoothly. 'Amazing Grace' might have appeared as a religious selection to those in the congregation, but it was a private joke between me and Michael. He had tried repeatedly to master the bagpipes and each time that he had worked on the chanter to perfect 'Amazing Grace', I seemed to be studying or researching. One day, after the usual, "Not now, Michael", he replied, "Well, Ma, I'll NEVER get to play 'Amazing Grace' for you, if I can't practice." He had sighed and given up, until one day he grinned and said, "Don't worry about it, Ma. If you go first, the organist can play that piece for you."

The song 'Clouds' had been requested by Anna and Bernie. That lyrical, romantic, yet profoundly sad piece certainly did represent Michael's life. When I heard the words of 'When You Walk Through a Storm', I shivered without control. I covered my mouth with a hankerchief so that I would not make a noise. Bruce had taken me to a presentation of Carousel while we lived in Hamilton. The first time I had heard that song, Michael had given me his initial quickening kick. It seemed to have such a special tie with him. Now it offered profound comfort.

When Bruce and I had entered the church, there had been less than a dozen people present. Two were friends of mine, who had lost a brother and a son from AIDS. I was grateful that they were present, because they alone comprehended our anguish. Somehow,

I had not expected many others to arrive. When the hymn was sung it seemed that a cloud of angels had settled over my shoulder, all singing lustily together. I listened in awe. Then, I realized that the church was filled with loving friends. We did not bid farewell to Michael in solitude. Compassion and understanding had banished loneliness. THANK YOU, GOD. THANK YOU.

The priest's homily provided spiritual edification, and afterwards, individuals praised his efforts to me. The readers lent a touch of elegance and astuteness. People had actually stood at the back of the church, due to the lack of sufficient seats. Afterwards, Bruce and I waited in a receiving line downstairs, before tables laden with the repast prepared by my sorority sisters. Sunlight streamed through the windows and kissed the many floral bouquets. OH, MICHAEL, THIS WAS A PERFECT TRIBUTE TO YOU.

Each meaningful gesture of sympathy soothed our ache. I recognized the large part played by the staff from my school within the ceremony. Michael's school chums passed by and hugged us. Amazingly enough, two architects who had studied with Michael in Europe shook our hands and promised to visit. Afterwards, Francine and her husband, with beloved neighbours, transported flowers, plants and left-over foods to our home. The day was completed, the service finished and we were tired to the bone. How grateful we were for the open support showered upon us. We had craved that healing! That night, for the first time since Michael's death, I slept soundly without medication. Contentment and exhaustion played their roles.

Two days later I returned to school to attend administrative meetings and complete year-end tasks. In my mail box was a sympathy card, containing a cheque for $1,000 from the staff. The money was to be used however I wished, to help defray some of the heavy costs of Michael's illness. I stood staring at it over and over, not quite believing the total. When I finally looked up, I saw the school secretaries gently smiling. I walked towards their desks, and said, "Did you see this? Incredible! Could I put it towards a school scholarship, in Michael's name? Do you think the Guidance Department could help me to do that, in time for graduation?" They assured me that it was feasible and it was established within an hour. The scholarship would be in Michael's name, in perpetuity. Graduation night I had the honour to present the first award on behalf of

NOT A TOTAL WASTE

Michael. As I passed that over to the selected student, I felt as though I had provided her with a gift from every staff member and Michael. It was an uplifting experience.

Cards and letters arrived from all over the world, to provide us solace in our loss. These have been re-read frequently. The Canadian Cancer Society and the Heart and Stroke Foundation expressed gratitude for numerous contributions made by friends.

We had planned to travel to Montreal to have Michael's urn buried in my husband's family plot, by the end of June. Our exhaustion eliminated that option. Michael's urn sits beside his enlarged photograph, on a long teak book case in our dining room. Bruce does not resent my reticence to part with Michael's remains, and I am grateful.

Exactly one week after Michael's memorial service, I contacted the priest to find out where he had hung the needlepointed tapestry of the Botticelli Madonna and Child. When he said that it was neither dedicated, nor hung, I arranged to meet him at the church that evening. To ensure completion of one more task, I brought along a hammer, hanging nails and the engraved memorial plaque. The priest expressed discomfort about the picture.

"I think that there really isn't any room for this art in the narthex, after all. And furthermore, this heavy gold frame doesn't match the light pine wooden walls. Maybe you could change the frame, or something."

"Father, don't you realize that the frame must match the piece of art? To change the frame would denigrate the value and appearance of the work. Father, you don't change the frame to match the wood in the hall--the frame must match the style of the art which it holds."

"I told you that I don't understand art. I don't have any idea where to hang it, nor do I have hammer and nails."

"I have them in the car, Father. I'll be right back. Perhaps you could determine an acceptable place to locate the tapestry, in the meantime."

"Not in the narthex. Not in the main church. Maybe in the stairwell here, or in the basement Sunday School area."

I did not respond, but went to get the plaque and tools. When I returned, he said,

"I've found the perfect spot. It can hang here and many people will notice it as they hang their coats."

"You mean that you want to hang it in the closet?"

"It's not exactly a closet. It has no door. It is an open section, where we hang our heavy winter coats all season. There's adequate lighting and room for the picture."

I stood very still, wondering about the efficacy of such a spot to hang this work. One of the parishioners entered the narthex. I handed her the tools to hang the picture and was too stunned to explain. The priest indicated the location to her, and together they hung the Botticelli--in the closet. I thanked the priest, took back the hammer and departed.

I lay my head upon the wheel of the car and pounded at the wheel with the palm of my hand. Struggling to control my emotions, I started slowly home. It seemed that the discrimination would never end, after all. I felt defeated and destroyed.

On the way home I purchased a cup of black coffee and returned to my car. I rolled the car windows down on that beautiful evening and sipped my beverage. Suddenly, I saw a strange aspect of humour to all of this. Michael had come OUT of the closet, but his memorial tribute would remain IN the closet. The zany side of me got a case of nervous giggles and I drank my coffee between laughter. If that's how the priest wanted it, so be it. I would just have to chuckle over it, secretly.

Three months later, the priest moved away. He had telephoned twice before that move, to ask if I required counselling, or wished to talk to him about my grief. He had sincerely offered help. A member of the congregation told me that the artwork was relocated to the back wall of the church, for all to enjoy. I have not yet returned to the church to see that for myself, but I plan to...someday, soon.

Struggling to obtain some measure of completion or healing after the death of a loved one is never a simple task. An AIDS Memorial Committee was formed in Toronto in 1988 with the goal of establishing a permanent tribute to all who have died of AIDS-related illnesses. In a treed area of Cawthra Square Park, behind the 519 Church Street Community Centre, within a few blocks of where Michael died, has been built a wall of names. Michael's name has been submitted for inclusion. The donation sent to defray any costs for adding his name to the wall was derived from an unusual source. It was earned by Michael posthumously from the publication of one of his own short stories, within the May 1992 Writers Supplement of Toronto's X-TRA paper.

In August of 1992, Michael's memorial quilt piece was completed and mailed to the Names Project of the AIDS Committee in Halifax, Nova Scotia. This three foot by six foot fabric piece will be incorporated along with the many other tributes to the lives of Canadians who have died of AIDS-related illnesses. My selection of the green linen background confirmed Michael's appreciation of that colour. Located among his private papers, was this unfinished short story which emphasizes his penchant for green:

"Somewhere in the distance a screen door bangs shut, the muted percussion section of a late summer evening. The freshly mown grass of the front yard is divided now into long streaks of forest green and emerald - emerald where the slanting rays of the sun slip between or over the houses and trees and lightly touch down, forest green where gathering shadows slumber.

My sister and I roll into a band of emerald on the northern edge of lawn that slopes down to our neighbour's drive, roll down and climb back up to roll down again. We squint against the low slung sun that steals between the houses, timid but insistent in its dying hour, squint as we clamber up the softly glowing bank.

If only money could be that colour. Then I would have a huge bank account, a solid abstraction of late summer evenings locked away knee deep in a cool steel vault, the numbers in my bank book telling of its ever growing depth. Then I would care about figures and multiplication, then I would care about financial stability and fiscal responsibility. But money is not that colour. No thing is that colour except freshly mown grass touched by the sun on a late summer evening. And so money, numbers, stability and responsibility mean nothing to me. I love only that colour. Nothing else.

It is a cool yellow-blue green with hints of darker blue beneath it and patches of gold hovering on its surface, hardly touching it, almost above it. It speaks of clean, dark pools hidden deep in forested valleys beneath a benevolent sky. It speaks of a gentle, dying heaven, a radiant old age that blankets with a loving caress even as it fades to make way for the cool blue that gathers beneath. And somehow, between the two, there emerges that wonderful emerald that fills up my soul and leaves room for nothing but the magic of this time, room for nothing but a shifting perfect present.

My sister and I tire of rolling and clambering on the slope, and lie on the band of light facing away from the sun into the gathering shadows of the distant horizon. We lie on our stomachs with our elbows out, pressed into the coolness of the grass. Our hands are clasped beneath our chins, our heads raised and casting long streaks of dark blue green into the vein of colour that stretches before us.

We lie there rearranging our legs, raising them now to shift the shape of the shadow beyond our heads, lowering them now into the first hints of the dampness that will be tomorrow's dew. The patterns before us grow longer, until suddenly the reflection of the sun flares from the window of our neighbour's house across the street and then vanishes over the roof into the gathering purple of the horizon. It is time to go in."

Sewn to the lower right corner of the quilt piece is a two foot by one foot cream linen section. This contains a glorious procession of crewel-embroidered summer field flowers, completed by my mother before her death fifteen years ago. Above that, chain stitched in four inch black letters upon the white fabric of one of Michael's well-worn pillow cases, is his name. To the left of that section is his photograph encased in clear plastic and a fabric frame made with left-over fabric swatches. The picture of Michael was taken for the Toronto Sun newspaper, when he was their SUNshine Boy. His golden hair is thick and unruly, his blue eyes mischievous, his body strong and healthy in his favourite blue jean outfit.

Beside the photograph are two appliqued squares of cross-stitched theatre masks of pathos and joy. His love of the arts made it applicable for me to complete those in his memory. Attached to the upper left section of the quilt is a fourteen inch square needlepointed butterfly on a cheery golden wool background. Michael chased and collected those lovely creatures throughout his childhood, but always set them free. While he studied at university he discovered an ancient Celtic tale about a priest whose spirit

NOT A TOTAL WASTE

entered a butterfly upon his death, in order to illustrate to his congregation that there was truly an afterlife. According to the story, the butterfly continues to represent the freedom of the spirit after death. Michael had enjoyed that tale. The background of the butterfly panel was completed in gold, because that was the colour of the comforting fog which appeared to me, against the ceiling of Michael's bedroom, upon his death.

Below the butterfly are sewn the dates of his birth and death, in black outline stitch on pieces of his white pillow case. Beside those dates is a cross-stitched square which reads, EXPECT MIRACLES and NOT A TOTAL WASTE. As much as possible, the memorial quilt piece is a jubilant celebration of many aspects of Mike's life, created with love. I look forward to seeing it incorporated with the other sections, when the quilt is next placed on tour.

In the back garden where Michael and Anna spent many hours playing with their dogs, Bruce has planted a beautiful Japanese cherry tree in Mike's memory. This spring and summer it blossomed and produced many small cherries. The wild birds have their feeder nearby, which Bruce keeps faithfully filled, but they also enjoy feeding upon the berries. That tree shall continue to grow, spread its limbs to provide shade and supplement the birds' diets. Michael would have approved.

CHAPTER SIX

During the first week in July, 1991, both of the grandchildren returned for their summer sojourn. They initiated their active schedule of swimming, sailing and skating activities. One night, after Jenni and Sean had completed their baths and shampooed the chlorine from their scalps, they sipped cool drinks at the kitchen table. Both children began to chat about their day's adventures.

"Turn off the light, Nana, light the candle and get the overhead fan going faster", suggested Jenni.
"May we also have some more ice cream, please, Nana?" questioned Sean.
"Sure thing. It sounds soothing, to me."
"Listen to the crickets, Nana."
"And the dogs barking back at them."

They giggled over that retort and seemed contented. They had used their roller-blade skates on the boardwalk down by the river that night and were showing sleepy signs of yawning and weary eyes. These special times, around the kitchen table together, were not unlike the reflective and restful evenings previously spent with their Mom and Uncle Michael as children. A strong bond had been formed with these precious grandchildren.

Jenni and Sean went into the dining room after their snacks were finished, on their way to give their Grampa his good-night hug. Sean stopped at the long teak bookcase, where Michael's photograph and urn remains. He looked at the photograph, reached out a tentative hand and then patted Michael's urn gently.

"Hi, Uncle Mike. How're you doing? I miss you..." Lovingly, Sean's hand stroked the picture frame and then both of his hands rested on top of the urn. I moved beside him and placed my hand on his shoulder. Large tears furrowed down his smooth cheeks, but he made no sound. His golden hair cascaded about his face in damp curls from his bath. His clear blue eyes searched mine, candidly.

"Oh, Sean, don't cry, dear. Uncle Michael wouldn't want you to be sad. Besides, I've cried enough for both of us."
"No, Nana. You don't understand. Me and Jenni have not finished our grief."

I turned and observed Jenni standing at the dining room doorway, her arms wrapped tightly across her chest, hugging her softly contoured little body. Auburn highlights shone from the tendrils of her shoulder-length hair, wispy against her cheeks. Her heart-shaped face was rigid and tense. Large, green eyes studied us cautiously.

"Nana, Sean's right. We didn't come to Uncle Mike's funeral. Mommy said that it was too far away."
"That's true. But Jenni, I would have sent tickets to fly you up. I just thought it was an unnecessary additional strain on both of you and Mommy, after all of that packing and unpacking of Uncle Michael's things. Your Daddy moved Uncle Michael every time that he had relocated himself at University. He has moved that furniture for the last time. You and Sean were both so brave when you helped me to get the urn from the funeral parlour in Toronto. Mommy was exhausted. I just thought...it seemed easier...to avoid any extra stress...and too far to have you travel. I'm sorry, kids. I guess that I was wrong. I wasn't thinking too clearly, at the time, and..."

Sean clenched his jaw, removed his hands from Michael's urn and turned to directly face me.

"It wasn't too far, Nana. We didn't get to say good-bye to Uncle Mike, like everybody else did. That wasn't fair."

Jenni nodded in agreement and moved around the dining room table to stand beside Sean.

"See Nana? We both feel the same. And did you really give the Botticelli tapestry to the church?"

"You remembered the name. My God...yes, I did."

"Why, Nana? Uncle Mike bought it for you, and you sewed on it for a long time."

"Well, it's called needlepoint, dear. It was dedicated at the church in Uncle Michael's memory."

"Does dedicated mean that you just gave it away?"

"It means that when people go to church to pray, they will take pleasure in its beauty. Then, they will remember Uncle Michael, too. When it hangs in the church, more people can see how beautiful it is, Jenni. It is a way of sharing, dear, with love and memories."

"Can we go and see it, Nana?"

"Certainly, Sean."

"But what about the other Madonna and child picture? The one that Uncle Mike said he liked a couple of years ago, when he came here."

"I don't know what you mean, Sean."

"Yes, you do. The other Mother and child. It's hanging in the frontroom, across from Grampa's chair. Uncle Mike said that he liked it, when he drove Mommy up here."

"Sean, that was over two years ago. I honestly cannot remember."

"Listen, it was the one that Uncle Mike said was very Byzantine. Now do you know the one I mean?"

"Byzantine? My God--you mean the Black Madonna tapestry, that Uncle Michael brought home from Europe for me."

"You sewed it too, Nana. It has got a heavy gold frame. How come it isn't at the church?"

"But, it would have to go to a Ukrainian or Greek Orthodox Church. That tapestry is very ancient, and copied from Byzantine-Kievan art work from the Eastern or Greek Empire of the fourteenth century. Uncle Michael said that he saw a copy in Poland. It is kept by the people of Czestochowa in a little wooden case, at the Monastery at Jasna Gora. There is a shrine on top of a hill. He said that it was a national relic connected with the Virgin Mary's life on earth."

"Do you know any more of the story, Nana?"

NOT A TOTAL WASTE

"Keep telling us what Uncle Mike said, please, Nana."

"Well, people apparently make pilgrimages from near and far to attend specific religious festivals, and they open the doors on the wooden case for the people to view the picture. Old stories, or legends say that it was dedicated to 'Our Lady, Virgin and Mother Mary', and that it was originally painted upon a wooden board. Uncle Mike told me that people believed that the wood was from the table top at which the Holy Family in Nazareth used to work and take their meals."

"That's weird, Nana. Maybe they were short of wood."

"No, Jenni. It's a way of showing love for Mary. And Jesus. It was their table--something left from them. Like when you hug Uncle Mike's teddy bear at night. Because it was Uncle Mike's, it makes you feel better, right?"

"Yes, Sean. But I sure would feel silly loving a table."

"It's a way of showing veneration, or affection, Jenni. Sean, they also say that when you look at the painting, the eyes follow you wherever you move."

"Uncle Mike's eyes do that, in the photograph that David took. Sometimes he smiles when I look at it, and sometimes he scowls. Mommy loves that picture."

"Well, now you know why the needlepointed picture is called a national relic. It is an important religious icon. That's all that I remember of Uncle Mike's explanation. Sean, I have no idea which local church would accept the Black Madonna tapestry."

"Nana, listen. Grampa showed us a new church up on the hill. It has golden onions on top. The picture should go there. We could take it."

"Those aren't onions, Jenni. Nana, she's dumb. Grampa said that they were domes. You should have paid attention. He told you they were domes, when we went for our drive."

"You mean the newly-built Ukrainian church. But, kids, I don't even know the priest at that church. I've never been inside. I can't just walk up and ask the priest to dedicate this tapestry for Uncle Michael."

"Why can't you? You gave the other picture to a church. Then we could have our own funeral. We could finish our grief."

"And Mommy said when we finish our grief, we'll feel better."

I stood, stunned and confused. Suddenly, both youngsters hugged me about my waist. Jenni wiped her nose against the back of her hand, sniffled and hugged me tighter. Sean patted my arm, walked into the front room and stood in front of the framed Black Madonna needlework, and said,

"I like it too, Nana. It's colours are bright and happy. It would be cheerful, in that new church. The reds and yellows and blues make me want to laugh. The Madonna is holding baby Jesus kindly. See how the gold frame matches the golden domes?"
"Domes do look like onions, Nana."

Jenni and I walked, stilted and awkwardly, towards Sean. We stared at the picture, together. Michael had brought that tapestry for me to needlepoint, from Europe. It was a beautiful piece, which I had thoroughly enjoyed completing. It provided the corner of that room with a richness, due to its depth of colour. I had used multiple weights of wool, and split numerous yarns to obtain the various colour-shading effects. Bruce had been sitting in his chair, monitoring this new development, without contributing any comments. Now he peeked overtop of his newspaper and said,

"It's time for bed, kids. Your swimming lessons begin early tomorrow morning. Say good-night now, and let Nana tuck you in. I'll come down in a few minutes to check on you both. Brush your teeth, too."

Silently the children turned towards him, looking surprised that he'd emerged from behind his newspaper and participated. Quietly, they nodded at one another, gave him a cursory peck on his cheek and started down the hall towards the bedrooms. I stood silently, contemplating this wondrous chain of events. How amazed I was that the youngsters could recall the exact art history terminology, after all that time. The words Byzantine, Botticelli, and domes had come easily to them. I started down the hall to determine whether the children had brushed their teeth, and were getting organized for their bedtime.

"Nana, did Mommy and Uncle Mike have goldfish when they were little?" Jenni sat on the edge of her bed, hugging Michael's teddy bear in her arms.
"Yes, Jenni. They had guppy fish, just like Grampa's, too. Your Mommy had a pet African frog called Angus, and it won first

prize in a pet contest. There was a picture of them in the newspaper. Angus grew as large as Grampa's hand and was constantly hungry."

"What other pets did they have? Did they have a big dog like ours?"

"Uncle Michael owned a pet snake, when he was your age. Grampa helped him search for its food, and they used to inspect the strange way that the snake engulfed its food. It pulls its jaws over the toad, gradually enwrapping it. Then it's body would show a round bulge, until the food became absorbed by its body. It ate little frogs, too, I believe. I couldn't stand to watch it eat, because the food had to be alive. The toads would go, "EEK" and I'd just shiver."

"Oh, yuck."

"Jenni, that's how wild animals are; they eat live things."

"You're right, Sean. They both had hamsters and cats and dogs, at one time or another. They also had a pair of yellow and green budgies, when they were very little children. Why, dear?"

"What happened to all of those pets, Nanna?"

"Well, I guess that they died."

"They got dead, just like Uncle Mike?"

"Yes."

"What did you do with their urns?"

"They didn't have urns, honey. We just buried them."

"Can we go and see their graves?"

"Jenni, I don't recall where they are located, after all of this time. I guess that some are buried in Hamilton, or Barrie, where we used to live. Some were probably buried in the bush across the street, before the new subdivision was built. Some were buried in the backyard, near all of the trees which Grampa planted. Two dogs' bodies were shipped to the University of Guelph, to be studied by other vets. They had cancer and heart disease which the doctors wanted to check out. That was a long time ago, dear."

"Did Mommy and Uncle Mike have a funeral for all of their pets?"

"For all of them? I really don't know. They showed me where they buried a hamster, once. It had popsicle sticks tied with wool, made into a cross, and lots of dandelion flowers on top of the little grave. Your Mommy and Uncle Mike planned the funerals, privately."

"Did they say a prayer to God?"

"Jenni, I don't know. Why?"

"Because little creatures have bodies. And they have souls. So we should pray for them, right?"

"I suppose so."

"Mommy says that we should."

"Then, you have the right answer. Of course."

"Daddy told me that you have to say good-bye when people die. That's why we went to Grampa Sam's funeral in London. Daddy was very sad, but he said he felt better after he helped to bury his father."

"Oh yes, that was last year."

"Nana, I miss my Grampa Sam. He made us laugh and he hugged us all the time. He could fix my bike and Mommy's freezer. Daddy used to drink cold beer with Grampa Sam and tell funny stories. We could jump on his tummy when he rested on the couch. Mommy said he was a good joker. We all loved him. Why did he have to die, Nana? He got so sick, like Uncle Mike. Will that happen to you and Grampa?"

"Well, honey, not for a long time, I hope. Everything dies some day. We're all dying, so I guess that we had better enjoy every single day. I know that you miss your Grampa Sam. He had a great sense of humour. Just try to remember all of the happy times. I try to do the same thing with my thoughts about Uncle Michael. Try not to be unhappy, dear."

"I am sad sometimes. Just like you are, Nana, when you talk about Uncle Michael and his sickness. Will my Mommy and Daddy die, too?"

"Some day, dear. Everybody eventually does die. But you're not to get upset about that, because Mom and Dad are young and healthy. They expect to be alive for a long time."

"Nana, Uncle Mike was young. Then he got sick."

"Well yes, honey, that's true."

"Daddy says that usually people's kids don't die before their parents. He says that its just not the right order for things."

"He's correct. We always expect that our children will live longer."

I looked up and realized that Sean was still standing at the bedroom door, holding his toothbrush in his hand and looking attentive. How had this conversation begun, when I had intended to tuck them into bed and kiss them good-night?

"Time out. Time out, you guys. No more death talk to-night, Nana. Please give us a backrub with that lotion, like you used to do last summer? Athletes love backrubs, you know."

"Sure thing, Sean. I have some cream on the top shelf of the linen closet. I'll fetch it, and finish Jenni's back first. Hurry to bed."

They slept deeply that night, but I didn't. Memories whirled around my head all night. I sat on the back porch with the dogs for awhile, sipping a mug of hot milk. Bruce found me there, around four o'clock.

"Don't you ever sleep?"

"The kids really threw me, this evening. Where do their ideas come from? One minute they are so old and wise and the next just little children, again."

"Yeh...a real challenge. What will you do, in order to achieve the closure they seem to need?"

"I can't imagine. I ought to talk it over with Anna and see if she has a solution. I don't feel too confident about discussing death and dying, right now. It's too damned close to me. Palliative care is easier if I'm not emotionally involved. This is tough stuff."

"Come to bed. You need rest."

The next morning, after Bruce had taken the children to their swimming lessons, we went for a hike. Bruce was determined that I should continue with some daily physical exercise to regain my physical stamina. He was certain that rest, good food, exercise, and fresh air would erase all vestiges of grief--and restore his wife to him. Even the smallest bit of exertion still left me drained. I couldn't run on nervous energy much longer.

Afterwards, we collected Jenni and Sean from their swimming lessons. We drove to the shopping mall to purchase new diving goggles, since the pool chlorine burned their sensitive eyes. While we window-shopped, a colleague stopped directly in front of us.

"Maria, I'm sorry about Michael's death. His loss is a tragedy. I hope that you won't be offended, but I have offered his name to our priest for a mass on Thursday evening. It's at the new Ukrainian church, on the hill. Will you attend?"

The children and I glanced quickly at one other, and stared at my friend.

"How thoughtful of you...may the children come, too?"
"Of course. I'll guide you through the service, if you wish."
"This is extremely kind of you!"
"Nothing to it. I am going to be talking with the priest today, and I'll request an English service, rather than Ukrainian, so that the children can follow along."
"Thanks."
"I'll call you later this evening, to confirm the time. Can you come, too, Bruce?"

Bruce smiled, but did not commit himself. Jenni clung to my hand, and Sean stood quietly beside me. Len kissed my cheek, squeezed my hand and was gone as quickly as he had apppeared. Jenni said,

"Come on, Nana. Let's get some O.J. or grape drink, okay, Grampa?"
Bruce nodded in agreement.
"Right on! Yeh, Nana and then we can talk", added Sean.
"That was peculiar, after all of that discussion last night. Will you dedicate the second tapestry?" asked Bruce.
"Now you got it!" replied Sean.
"Great idea, Grampa!" exclaimed Jenni.

I knew when I was beaten. This strange chain of events must not be without a purpose. That afternoon, I had a bronze memorial plaque engraved in Michael's memory. I packed it with the tapestry in the car and drove to the church on the hill. When I entered the vestibule in search of the priest, I marvelled at the proliferation of beautiful paintings which hung in the inner church and the foyer. Soft lighting emanated from the curved ceiling, giving a subdued glow to the white walls. It was truly a beautifully-designed house of worship. After chatting with the priest, I offered a cheque towards the mass for Michael, to be held on Thursday. Then, I put forth my request.

"Father, would you please take a look at a needlepoint, which I have completed and framed, for the church? My son brought it back from Europe for me. It is a Madonna and child tapestry. If you approve of it, would you consider it as a memorial tribute for my

NOT A TOTAL WASTE 255

son? I have it, and a bronze engraved plaque, in my car. It would not matter to me, where you hung it. Your office, or the basement..."

"You mean that you would like me to dedicate it on Thursday? Why, of course. Let me see it."

I retrieved the tapestry from the car, unwrapped it and offered it for the priest's inspection. He accepted the large art work and held it carefully in his hands. His eyes filled with sudden, unexpected tears. I watched his reaction with surprise.

"But...it is the Black Madonna...it is a Ukrainian Icon. We don't have a copy of it within our church. You have completed a beloved liturgical artifact. It is truly magnificent. THANK YOU! It is a treasure!"

"Then, you won't mind dedicating it in Michael's memory?"

"It will be an honour. This art will hang inside the church, on the back wall where it can be seen and enjoyed by everyone."

"Within the church, proper?"

"Yes, definitely. We'll dedicate it during the service. Thank you most sincerely for this exquisite work. We shall value it. We look forward to seeing you and your two grandchildren at seven, on Thursday. Len has explained the need for an English mass celebration."

I smiled, nodded and left. "Well, I'll be damned," I thought to myself. I remained transfixed in my car for a few moments, comparing this experience of the needlepointed Madonna and child, with the prior Botticelli donation. How incredible this event seemed. What a contrasting attitude this priest had exhibited, upon receipt of the Byzantine tapestry.

On Thursday, I dressed the children in new outfits and wore the white linen suit which I had used for the memorial service. Bruce was reading the newspaper when Jenni urged him to hurry. I grinned at him when he muttered that Jenni refused any negative response. His only choice was to attend. Just before our departure, Len phoned to explain that in lieu of any other names put forth for the celebration of mass that evening, the priest was prepared to offer a complete funeral liturgy in Michael's honour. I kept that development secret, and continued to monitor their progress towards the car.

Upon our arrival, Len escorted us to the front pews, and supplied the required texts. Only a dozen other people were present. With beauty and sensitivity, the priest and his attendant conducted the ceremony, wearing exquisite golden robes, crisp white vestments and crimson cummerbunds. Sean whispered to me that they were dressed in "Byzantine outfits", and I agreed. The children both paid careful attention to the entire service, and followed Len's lead in kneeling or standing. The priest sprinkled holy water on the tapestry and sang the dedication.

Upon hearing Michael's name mentioned within that part of the ceremony, tears flowed unimpeded down the children's faces. They followed all aspects of the service meticulously. When I was remiss, they patiently whispered corrections. Afterwards, they walked sedately down the aisle towards the priest and his assistant.

"Thank you, Father," Sean said, offering his hand to the priest. "You really helped me to finish my grief. Some of the hurt is gone, now. I feel better."

Jenni walked up to the priest, curtsied, and said, "Father, thanks a lot. I feel better, too. I'm glad that the picture is dedicated, now. It sure looks good there."

I shook the priest's hand, too, and murmured my appreciation. This had not been a doleful ceremony, but a very formal, religious experience. However, I couldn't say much, because my throat was restricted from emotion. The actions of the children had been natural and graceful, without prior instruction. Despite the small congregation, it had seemed as if numerous angels had provided a chorus. I stumbled down the aisle after Jenni and Sean, grateful for Bruce's hand supporting my elbow. He steered me towards the car, patted my hand and helped me into the vehicle. Our eyes met, and held. He smiled gently, with eyes filled. We felt warmed with love, and at peace. Once we were all buckled into the car seats, Jenni sang out happily,

"Okay, Grampa, move your buns! We're going to Tim Horton's donut shop."
"We are? How come?"
"Grampa, BECAUSE. This is Uncle Michael's day. He loved donuts when he wasn't sick. You remember, the kind that you squeeze, and strawberry jam squishes out. So, aw-a-y we go. Donuts and cocoa, here we come!"

NOT A TOTAL WASTE

"Yay--good idea, Jenni. Is that all right with you, Nana and Grampa?"

Bruce looked at me, and I saw that he was fighting back emotion. He cleared his throat, blinked and concentrated on getting the car started.

"Of course, kids. I'm glad that you two reminded me to come and share this evening."

"We are too, Grampa. Because--you have to pay the bill!"

We laughed together and commenced our trip.

Once the children were tucked in for the night, I called Anna to describe our amazing experiences of the last few days. However, when I started to describe the "second funeral" and the "second dedication", she got extremely agitated.

"Why did you do this to my children? They didn't need to go through all that emotional carnage. Why can't you just let Michael go? Whose idea was this, Mom?"

"It just...sort of happened. I guess I am to blame."

"And the second tapestry being dedicated? Whose idea was that? Was that your idea, too?"

"I'm...to blame...for all of it, Anna."

"Michael's dead, Mom. Face it. I never should have sent the children this summer. It's too soon. You could do a lot of damage with your damned sorrow. He's dead, Mother. Michael is DEAD. It's over. Let him go."

She hung up. I winced and sat in shock, not even able to weep. My body felt icy cold. I shivered and trembled. I hated the power of that violent shaking, which left me without any control. It had been that way when I was alone, in Michael's apartment, after his death. Now, those same sensations had returned. I stumbled as I stood and then numbly wandered down the hall. I bounced off the art work which hung on the walls along the way, until I reached my bed. I had not intended to hurt the children emotionally. I hoped, desperately, that they were unaffected. The church service had not been maudlin. It had stressed the spirituality of birth and death. So much intrinsic beauty and power surrounded both of those life experiences.

Anna was right, all the same. These were not my children, but were only left in my trust for the brief month of July. I should not have proceeded with the ceremony, without her permission. I was immersed in the throes of anguish once again. How I could have discerned such an elation--only to become crushed again, so rapidly? Why wouldn't this pathos be alleviated? How could it return and overwhelm me like this? Anna's anger had cut me to the quick. Because of my stupidity, had I lost Anna, too? First Michael...now Anna...PLEASE GOD, NO! Without Michael, I fought against my instinct to overprotect Anna--to pull her too tightly to my heart. Alone, I tried to cope with a dejection that bore through to my very soul. Anna had been hurt by my thoughtless neglect to seek her permission. She was also grieving, in her own way and at her own pace. Sibling grief produced unique stresses. Old rivalries surfaced and many wounds reopened. I appealed to God for strength, wimpered into my pillow and fitfully slept.

CHAPTER SEVEN

The first Friday in August, Bruce and I returned the grandchildren to their parents in Hamilton. They were taller, tanned, healthy and eager to see their folks and friends. When Anna met our plane at Terminal III, we all hugged and kissed. Bruce and I departed immediately in a limousine to the Downtown Holiday Inn on Chestnut Street. After contacting his octogenarian mother, Bruce left to spend the evening with her.

Isolated in the hotel room, I looked out of the window from the sixteenth floor upon the vista of Toronto's unique City Hall. It was shaped like two giant sea shells, facing one another. Around the corner strolled a young man, wearing a jacket similar to Michael's, heading towards the hotel. Unprompted, my mind initiated a visual narration of past visits spent with Michael.

A jumble of reminiscences overlapped in confusion, devoid of logical sequence. His smiling face and contagious laughter changed quickly, in my mind's eye, from a youthful, exuberant student to a wan, frail invalid. He refused either cane or wheelchair, and lurched in an ungainly manner towards me. With mounting hysteria, I realized that it was too soon for me to be in Michael's Toronto, alone. My chest felt caught within the jaws of a steel vise, which persistently tightened until I swore that I could not breath. I was terrified.

I staggered towards the bed, and concentrated on breathing out, with only small inward gasps. I needed carbon dioxide, not extra oxygen. Gradually, my fear abated. I inhaled and exhaled cautiously. Obviously, it would take me longer than I had anticipated to face a Toronto visit, without engendering painful memories which engulfed reality. I closed my eyes and concentrated on regulating my breathing.

The telephone rang at 6:30, and Bruce suggested that I order room service for dinner, since his visit with his mother would detain him. When I hung up the phone, it rang immediately. This time, it was David.

"Hi there, Maria. I just checked with Anna, since Kim was almost certain that you'd be bringing Jenni and Sean home this week-end. She told me where you are staying. How are you doing?"

My eyes misted and I gripped the telephone receiver.

"David! How thoughtful of you to remember. I'm okay...some bad times...some good times."
"Well, can you meet me and Kim for dinner this evening?"
"No, David. I'm afraid not."
"Bring Bruce! He'd be very welcome."
"He's visiting his mother."
"Get a taxi. Just come over for a brief visit and have a glass of champagne. Come on now--at least you can give us that much of your time. We won't accept no for an answer. See you in half an hour."
"That would be truly pleasant. See you soon."

I showered, changed, hailed a cab and arrived at David's lovely Rosedale home by 7:30. He politely refrained from mentioning my swollen, reddened eyes or haggard appearance. David, his friends and I shared a quiet drink of French champagne, and chatted. The background music was Mitsuko Uchida's recording of Mozart's Sonata in C, K. 279, right through to Eine Kleine Gigue in G, K. 574. The exquisite clarity of the music, and the pleasant conversation were soothing. By nine o'clock, I was back at the hotel and asleep when Bruce returned.

NOT A TOTAL WASTE

The next day, we sauntered through the Eaton's Centre and window shopped. There was little pleasure to this hike. On the contrary, it left me agitated. Michael and I had spent so much time walking in these same places. Once his illness caused him to sleep from fourteen to sixteen hours a day, I had sipped coffee near the fountain, alone and despondent. I recalled shared chats with Michael at Biffy's Bistro, that special lunch at the Queen Mother Cafe and strolls through the University of Toronto campus. Many high teas shared with David and Michael at the King Edward and the Windsor Arms rushed through my mind.

It seemed as though I met Michael's image at every corner, and a rising panic threatened to overwhelm me. I begged Bruce to get me back to the hotel. The strength of those surrealistic images left me shaken. The power of my subconscious was potent with visions of Michael. When we flew back home the next morning, we busied ourselves with tasks around the house. For a few weeks we tackled hikes each morning and tried to unwind. Bruce's health-kick regime left me exhausted, but more relaxed.

A week before school started, I was determined to duplicate lesson plan materials for the first week of classes. I headed towards the school but, without warning, was forced to pull off the highway. Tremors shook my body again, and tears blinded my vision. The car radio played Glenn Gould's Bach--The Goldberg Variations--which Michael had enjoyed. Almost immediately, I could heaar Mie's voice speaking to me as clearly as if he sat beside me. "Listen, Mom. Gould's HUMMING. His mother tutored him from childhood. She instructed him to warrrble softly, in order to maintain a measured tempo. Its amazing! His brilliant pianist skills and his amusing vocal trills were recorded for eternity." A smile tugged at the corners of my mouth. Michael had been delighted at that absurd correlation of cadence and cacophony. I had come to the section of the highway where Michael had helped me to learn to drive the car. Even though I had taken lessons from a driving school, it had been Michael who had patiently practiced me on highway travel. I yearned to hear his voice and see his smile.

I realized that I could not go to school in this state, so when I had recovered sufficiently I drove directly to the medical clinic. I requested an emergency appointment with my doctor and his office nurse arranged for me to see him quickly.

"Looking at your chart, you haven't been here for awhile. What seems to be the problem, Maria?"

"Well, I guess I've been dealing with a type of panic or anxiety attack. It's hard to explain. But...I need your help. Thought I could do this by myself. Looks like I can't."

"This is unlike you. Give me some details. Talk to me."

"Our only son died in June. I was sure that I had a handle on this. I believed that I was coping. Well, school starts on Monday. I'm scared. I can't face this pressure. Please...can you give me some type of medication to keep me calm, so that I won't cry and act like a nut case?"

"Ummhmm. About your son. How old was he?"

"Only thirty-three. Too young. My best friend. For some reason, this grief is more torturous than I expected."

"What did he die from? Was he sick long?"

"Well...I tell everyone it was cancer. Because...he did have cancer everywhere. He was partially paralyzed from brain lesions. They were in his throat, lungs, abdomen..he was severely dehydrated. It was an AIDS-related death. Michael was ill for two years, but most especially during the past year."

"You knew, once he was diagnosed, that he would die."

"Sure, but I denied it. I hoped that with luck, he would still have a few more years. Or even one more year. I kept hoping they'd find a cure. Mike teased me because I expected miracles."

"And now he's dead."

"Yes. I don't use any euphemisms, like 'passed on', or 'gone away'--he's just dead. It sounds so bloody final."

"It is final. How are you handling your grief?"

"I can't. It comes over me in waves, when I least expect it. Just when I think I'm adjusting well--something triggers it, and I've lost any control. It could be an oreo cookie or an adult diaper advertisement. I can't predict when I am going to fall apart. I'm weepy and ashamed of my weakness."

"Maria, you can't intellectualize emotion. No-one can do that. You're being awfully hard on yourself. Can you talk with your husband, Bruce, about this anguish?"

"He hates to see me upset. He says, 'Knock it off'. He asks, 'When is this going to be over?' He's into denial, and has experienced difficulty in coping throughout the past two years. He did not communicate with Michael once he knew that he was terminally ill. This whole thing creates excruciating grief. I thought I understood loneliness before, but..."

"I see. Have you both considered counselling?"
"Please, we don't want that. Maybe later. We just cannot open up to a stranger. We can't even discuss Mike rationally with each other. It's especially difficult..."
"Because your son died of AIDS? You realize, don't you, that such a death will make it considerably tougher for you to complete your bereavement? While you are battling to protect your confidentiality, you will not grieve normally. You will remain on the defensive, and it will be a higher wall for you to breach."
"Grieve normally. Or abnormally. I'm not sure if there is such a big difference between chronic grief and what I am experiencing. I guess that I am acting defensively. Closets are for clothes, or little kids' toys. Mike was 'out of the closet', but I must remain circumspect. I act warily and I'm frightened. I have the responsibility of thirty different students every hour of the day. I can't possibly disintegrate in front of my classes--I'm expected to cover essential curriculum content. It's futile, without help."
"Are you familiar with the local AIDS support network? Apparently, they are doing a fine job assisting families."
"Yes. I was a part of the initial group. My friends are taking care of all that, and I am not prepared to get involved now."
"I see. Have you had alprazolam tablets before? You dislike taking any medication, but these are only 0.5 mg, so they are fairly mild. In fact, I'll give you a prescription for an additional mild tablet, ativan sublingual, also only 0.5 mg. You try the sample of alpraxolam, and decide which medication you prefer. The prescription is essentially a light anxiety-reliever. Maria, you have to realize that what you are experiencing, is not abnormal."
"I don't want the pills, if they are addictive."
"You know me better than that. I wouldn't let you take anything that was addictive. I'm only giving you thirty, and if you need more, you will have to see me to discuss how you're coping."
"You know that I am not going to take them regularly. I'll only use them when it is an emergency situation."
"Yes, I know how independent you are about medication. Now, if these don't do the job, come back to see me. Don't just wallow around like a lost soul. Get back to me. Sorrow is difficult-- but yours is more complicated. You see, social alienation can increase the impact of grief. Therefore, it is potentially risky for your health."
"I thought that I was cracking up. I despise this lack of control."

"You'll be better, Maria. You just can't rush it. You survived the past two years. You had to be strong to manage throughout Michael's illness. Was he brave, too?"

My eyes filled quickly and I couldn't swallow. I simply nodded. The doctor patted my shoulder and said gently,

"Losing your only son is one of the most devastating things for a mother."
"It feels as though half of me is gone. Torn from me. Forever."
"Part of you IS gone. He will not come back. You can't fix it. However, he'd want you to be as courageous as he was--and to regain your strength."
"I know. Michael wouldn't want me to be this morbid. This inconsolable."
"It's still very soon, since his death. How is your sleeping ability?"
"Lousy."
"Eating?"
"Everything tastes like straw. I either overeat for comfort, not even aware of what I am eating, or I go without food. Cooking smells make my stomach heave."
"Are you exercising?"
"Yes. Light stretching exercises and short hikes."
"Have you been doing any research related to grief?"
"Oh, I must have read over sixty books. Nothing helps. They all stop at the death, as if the world is wonderful after that. There are books about the loss of babies, little children, old parents, husbands, wives and pets. Nothing about the loss of an only, mature son. Nor do they explain this particular kind of loss. AIDS is such a messy combination of so many diseases."
"How is your husband managing?"
"He seems okay. He won't talk about it."
"Was he helpful to you?"
"He has done what he can."
"You were essentially the main care giver?"
"Yes, with assistance from my daughter, and some of Michael's friends. I couldn't have managed without them."
"Can you keep in touch with Michael's friends?"
"I do. We telephone and write, and I contact them when I am in the city. But it's not fair for me to depend upon them. They're struggling with grief and worries for their own futures. More than

NOT A TOTAL WASTE

one of them has tested HIV positive. They are precious links to many special memories of Michael. I've grown to respect and love them, too. I can't help worry about them, as well...but the last thing that they need is an emotive, old mother pestering them. I try to wait until they contact me first."

"Will the marriage relationship improve, do you think?"

"We just both have to mourn in our own way, I guess. It's going to take awhile. Is it true that time will heal this bloody ache?"

"Maria, you will never relinquish that trauma. It won't go away. You will always have times when the memories will rush in and take over. All that I can tell you is that eventually you'll learn to adapt to your sorrow. As you recognize which events trigger your emotions, you'll work through that anguish. In the meantime, you have to learn to take care of yourself, and to be good to yourself, too."

The doctor patted my shoulder, reminded me to call him if I needed him, and I left to fill the prescription. I was grateful for his consideration--and the security which the pills would provide. Until I recovered my strength, they would serve as a panacea for the pain, a cathartic crutch to keep me standing.

CHAPTER EIGHT

Once school began in September, I attempted to keep myself so active that I wouldn't have time to dwell upon Michael's death. Certainly, being at school with the young people was comforting. Their effervescence and vitality were contagious. Besides lesson preparations, research, teaching and marking, little time remained for maudlin morbidity.

However, I also undertook additional professional obligations, as a means of generalized withdrawal from the mainstream of society. My efforts to escape from my own thoughts resulted in a driven hyperactivity. Whereas some individuals might have employed alcohol or drugs to avoid past-oriented thoughts, I lost myself in over-work. I avoided seeking additional support services, because I still felt overwhelmed by Michael's loss. Work was my refuge.

Because I still resisted offers of support from my network of friends or loved ones, I also avoided taking the prescribed medication from my doctor. The one month's supply of anti-anxiety pills was still not depleted by the end of six months. Coping procedures were relied upon, only as last ditch methods for survival. Perhaps my anger kept me functioning, more than I realized at the time. Bruce was blamed for any lack of affection between us, despite my refusal to respond to any overture. In contrast to my caution not to

NOT A TOTAL WASTE

over-idealize Michael, I frequently belittled Bruce's sincere efforts at strengthening our marriage. I responded with indifferent ambivalence.

Furthermore, I harboured frustration that Michael's doctors had not aggressively treated him for complex bowel infections. I kept remonstrating that they should have tested more prodigiously for a nutritional supplement to nourish his weakened, thin body. Resentment against society accumulated because of the inadequate medical treatment proffered for AIDS-related illnesses. The international snubbery for evidence of the catastrophic spreading of AIDS among the heterosexuals throughout the third world countries left me infuriated. Michael had spoken of his concerns often, since women in such poverty-ridden countries are politically powerless to insist upon the use of condoms. Promiscuity has been touted as the major propagator of African Aids. In addition, there has been virtually no medical screening of blood in diverse sections of the Third World. Asia has been referred to as the sleeping giant of this worldwide epidemic. The AIDS plague could devour many innocent third world women and children before society would heed the statistics.

I felt fury towards Bruce, Michael's doctors, and society's disdain. My rage seemed aimed at the world in general, and I tortured myself with many "I should have done's", as well. Somehow, I had absorbed and experienced every torment which Michael had endured, and blamed myself for my inability to prevent his demise.

It was not until one year after Michael's death that both Anna and I took anonymous HIV tests, to ensure that we would not purposely cause our loved ones injury. Our results were negative. We learned of a new disease which resembled AIDS, but which could not be discerned in the blood. Perhaps Mike's concerns of a mutating AIDS virus had some factual base. However, a global quest for artificial blood has created competition among hemoglobin scientists. A synthetic blood that could be easily stored, could be transfused into people of any blood type and would be guaranteed free of blood-borne diseases such as hepatitis and AIDS, would prove to be a miracle. Anna and I can only hope that the apparent lack of any HIV virus within our blood tests indicated that we were free of the disease.

Researchers persisted with their work on dozens of experimental vaccines. By June of 1992 the third drug, DDC, was finally approved for use by the U.S. Food and Drug Administration. However, the predictions of an evolving epidemic of AIDS among heterosexuals and children throughout the world continued to climb. The deadly microbe scoffed at scientists. Elizabeth Taylor was quoted in the August 1992 TIME magazine (page 20) as stating that, "Now is the time for global solidarity against a common enemy. Now is the time for us to share our knowledge." Would the world listen and repond? Would they react in time to stem a major loss of lives? When I surveyed past events, Michael's medical team had done their decisive best, Bruce had provided proper assistance, and my own efforts had been all that I had to offer. Still, international societal response lagged dangerously.

My personal continuum of bereavement responses drained my health, and left my immune system affected. I battled cysts scattered throughout my body, including fibrocystic breast disease related to the onset of the menopause. Deep vein thrombosis in my leg created discomfort and concern that the clots would move throughout the body. Mild exercises were employed to rebuild my stamina. Migraines strained my eyesight, and made relaxation difficult. There were recurring emotional "crazy" spells, triggered by events of the past. Sleep patterns were altered drastically. I slept for two to four hour periods, and then wandered aimlessly about the house. During those restless sessions, I undertook mundane menial tasks, read, or watched late-night television to exhaust myself. The impact of stress created short-term memory losses. Names, dates, and destinations confused me. Food either held no interest, or I "pigged out" because I felt depressed.

Socially, I withdrew as much as possible. I selected special, safe friends to visit, and never chose the same person twice. Efforts to communicate with Bruce remained complicated. Either I remained aloof, or tried too hard to define my personal emotional upheaval and was accused of oral diarrhea. Bruce rejected my pain, since he was undergoing his own trauma, escalated by the impact of an uneasy retirement. I avoided crowds, unless I possessed some manner of control--such as instructing within the university or secondary school classroom. Recreational outlets were also rationed cautiously. Although I had maintained my membership, I was too drained to proceed with an excerise routine at the fitness

NOT A TOTAL WASTE

club. The sensation that my heart was bound tightly with barbed wire, was eventually less excruciating.

To outsiders, my countenance appeared fairly poised and calm. I truly enjoyed teaching, but exhaustion was a genuine hazard. By caring for my students' needs, and by keeping myself active every minute of every day, no brooding time remained. The work load which I had undertaken was brutal. Overfatigue left me vulnerable and tearful. Desperately, I avoided my own sorrow by forcing myself to be oriented to the present moment.

Repetitive thoughts persistently intruded during quiet times. An appropriate curb on my feelings and thoughts was retained publicly. When I over-extended myself and depleted my strength, weepy, uncontrolled crying sessions filled my solitudes. Nostalgic memories crowded my mind during any restful interlude. Through a piecemeal process, I obliterated some of the anguish and acknowledged my gratitude for the genuine privilege of having known and loved Michael.

By focussing on the meaning and impact of Michael's life and death, I began to experience less anger at his loss, and more appreciation for having shared his life. Step-by-step, the periods of discouragement and helplessness decreased. With effort, I gradually began to accept the reality of Michael's death. In a world devoid of his friendship and love, I struggled to reinvest my strength, energy and skills in my marriage, Anna and her family. Michael had left behind a legacy of courage, integrity, intelligence and affection. His life had been an example of nonjudgemental acceptance and compassion for others who suffer.

Michael's committed concern for the environment, for future economic global ties, for retraining and educating society, for eliminating illiteracy, for the dispersion of any kinds of discrimination, provided lifetime goals. Those emotions and intimacies experienced during Michael's last remaining days had acutely developed sensitivity to my surroundings, caution against setting restrictive goals and responsiveness to individual needs. By knowing and loving Michael, I acquired an expanded empathy and sensitivity. I hope that his love has made me a better person.

I cannot say that I have ascertained any real meaning in Michael's death. Somehow, I survive without him. However, there is considerable value in the life which he has lived. Cherishing him has irrevocably changed me, and will affect any subsequent loving relationship. Those unpredictable and lonely times of my grief created frightening feelings and behaviours which were haunted, helpless and hurtful. Such interludes cannot be erased, but I have attempted to prepare myself for anticipatory emotive cycles. That first Christmas after Michael's death impacted upon all of his loved ones. His birthday and the anniversary of his death will always be recognized as significant occasions.

Michael's friends have persistently reached out their hands with affection and caring. Brief visits, phone calls and letters from Corey, Ted and Laura have been delightfully filled with laughter and nostalgia. Highlights of every business trip to Toronto have included dinner parties with David and Kim. Flowers, cards and letters have recounted great experiences which Michael's friends had shared with him throughout his lifetime.

Considerable comfort is derived from Michael's belongings. He feels nearby when I wear his special birthday shirt, or listen to his cassette tape of Ivo Pogorelich's recording of Beethoven's Piano Sonata no. 32 in C minor. When I languidly browse through his eight photograph albums, Michael smiles at me from diverse corners of the world. Sorting through his art portfolio impacts upon my senses, powerfully. His own life values and aspirations for being a productive member of society have not been obliterated, but will remain a tangible part of my very being. I am endeavoring to forgive myself for my inability to prevent his death.

I recognize the fact that I will never completely adapt to losing Michael. Grieving simply continues each day, since it is not a passive experience. However, increased periods of peacefulness have permitted me to muse over some humorous anecdotes, recall special moments, or reminisce without anguished yearning. I laughed outright while listening to Michael's voice, discovered on two humorous tape recordings among his music collection. The following letter, written November, 1985 from Japan, was relocated when I tidied up a drawer in November, 1992. It effectively expressed how truly Michael wanted to live productively, and with love.

NOT A TOTAL WASTE

Dear Ma,

As there has been a fairly lengthy gap in communication, and as I am curious as to how you are doing, I have decided to MAIL YOU A LETTER! WOW!

It's a blustery, sunny autumn day. All the leaves are down on the Kaki tree in the back yard, though the persimmons do not appear to be ripe yet, and none of the other trees have even begun to change colour yet. However, some of the maples on the hills have changed. I expect you are all knee-deep in snow by now. At least you'll have a white Christmas.

I have still not started my Japanese lessons. My schedule is just a wee bit up in the air still, and until it gets settled there is really no way to arrange for lessons. I am surviving by using pidgin English, pointing and miming (AND pretending I don't live here, to save face).

Egon is going to Europe for 2-3-4 months (Egon is the Austrian who rents the house) so we have to try to find someone else to take over for him in his room, to keep utilities down. Maybe. (i.e., heating costs, which may turn prohibitive). For now, I have Ginger, the house cat, keeping me warm, and my sweatshirts and the sunshine. The fact that it is only cool, not cold, and my hot cup of barley tea are additional assets.

I have meat balls and spaghetti sauce burbling merrily away on the stove. I have been eating a lot of pasta again (I get in these pasta moods...) and it has become a bit of a joke here. Some Japanese food is quite edible. Some of it is just plain appalling! But it's low in fats, so good for your heart, etc...Too much boiled stuff, though. BORING! I could use a good meat pie. I'll have to go out and pick up a pie plate. Does Anna have a recipe for meat pie? YUM! I just tried one of my meat balls. I think I'd better bring in my laundry before it blows away down the hill (there is about a 10 metre vertical drop from our back yard to the house below) to be lost forever.

There is no one here but me. I like it best like that. Alone, to watch the sun gild the furniture and the wind bend the trees. I can play whatever music I want, as loud as I want, and I don't have to entertain anybody, or pretend to like them when I'm not in the mood to like them. I'm turning into at least as much of a loner, as you two. I wonder if it has something to do with the fact that I've been working with people so much. When I was architecting, staring at a drafting board all day, I was forever going out and trying to engage people in conversation. Since I started waitering and teaching, I've lost that urge. I'm not totally antisocial, but I am no longer out there aggressively seeking human companionship. Is it just 'cuz I'm getting "olde"? I think I'm finally growing up folks (I know we've waited long enough for this). I'm so much calmer now than I was three years ago. I'm not trying to prove anything anymore. (At least, not nearly so much, and I think not in a negative way).

The turning point came in Edmonton, of course, one night on the high level bridge, in 1981. Then there was that day in Rome, when the Christian work ethic (God knows where that had come from) bit the dust, and I decided not to work because it was "morally right to produce" and be "the best worker I could be" but rather to work at something that I WANTED to do and would ENJOY doing, and to keep food on the table and a roof over my head (and maybe the odd dinner out, and maybe that new sweater, and maybe...). Materialistic little bugger, ain't I? That moment (in the studio bar in Rome) finished architecture as a life. To be an architect, architecture must BE your life. It took me a bit longer to reach that point in Rome than it takes most people, because I was effectively paralyzed from about 16 or 17 till 22 or 23 by what became, by the ages of 19, 20, 21, 22, an increasingly complete suicidal mentality, which you may or may not have noticed when I was still living at home.

As I'm sure you know, I had always been conscious of being extremely different from most people (because I always was). Not just in terms of sexuality, but in numerous other ways as well. I was always distant, and fairly (?!understatement?!) abstracted. Anna taught me the necessity of "fitting in" towards the end of grade seven, when the physical bullying at school had reached absurd proportions. I was simply an arrogant self-righteous little bugger, using that behaviour to cut off my sense of inferiority (physical, only) and my growing awareness (even then) of my sexual interests. So, I learned to "fit in".

NOT A TOTAL WASTE

It wasn't easy, and the fact that it was never sincere didn't help matters. However, I ceased to be insufferable to the group. This nonetheless set up a rather fearful dichotomy between my real self and my "stage" persona which, combined with an active and cold mind (it can be quite cold when it comes to questions of pure logic) set up a basic problem with accepting anything as "real".

Therefore, I embarked on an inquiry into the nature of reality (at the age of 12). Of course, I got swamped. As I was not a deeply religious man, I had none of the religious bars against suicide, and as the world appeared more and more meaningless, and my life less and less purposeful (and meaning and purpose were extremely important to me) and as I became increasingly conscious of the impossibility of ever really fitting social norms or fulfilling the racial (to do with species) notions of family, reproduction, house and home and wife and kids--romantic, lasting love with one person (male or female) till death do us part (I ceased to believe in the possibility of this concept being true around 21), I became increasingly cynical and divorced from the world. And, of course, suicidal.

When life becomes utterly devoid of meaning and purpose, the daily struggle (however feeble, or however easy that struggle should be) becomes a bit much. This, of course, culminated in a series of suicide attempts, none of which came to much. The closest I got was when I was actually quite young--16--and I swallowed a bunch of pills. I did everything possible after swallowing them to keep myself alive--push ups, running, throwing up, but I was still very sleepy for a few days. I didn't trouble you with it at the time, because you couldn't have helped--nobody could. Neither physically (I had tossed 90% of what I had taken) nor emotionally. That, I had to settle on my own.

After a number of less dramatic attempts, but in the face of increasing desperation, I found myself one night on the high level bridge in Edmonton, pondering the jump. This was after I had dropped out of architecture for the first time, when my mental state made continuing utterly impossible (Its very hard to interest yourself in something when you're not sure you'll be there the next day). I had just accepted the fact that I would never find anyone to love "til death do us part" and had therefore abandoned my last reason to live (not much of a reason, anyhow).

However, I found that I quite simply didn't WANT to jump, that, just as when I was 16, my will to live was stronger than my suicidal impulse, even though I could find no rational reason to live. This amazed me. There was no reason at all to live that I could perceive rationally, but, there I was, I had EVERY INTENTION of living. I went over the other times I had considered suicide, attempted it (almost invariably half-heartedly) and decided, empirically, that I was not going to commit suicide, that I had a wholly irrational but effectively ABSOLUTE DESIRE TO LIVE. So much for Descartes. Empirical reason was something new in this context, and the conclusion was a revelation.

From that point, I started taking an interest in life--from that point I started paying attention, started growing up. Of course, I didn't get better all at once. I was still a mess for a couple of years. But at least I had accepted the fact that I was going to live and that I had better start making some plans that would last longer than a day or two (real plans, not sham plans for public consumption). Its amazing how things suddenly take on depth and start making sense when you stop dealing with abstract ideals and get about the business of living. I started looking at things in a whole new way once I had decided that I was, in fact, going to be here, and not just tomorrow, but for some time. From this point on I started to make up for lost time. I had lost so much, though. That's why I've taken so long to grow up. Sorry about the delay. It has been very interesting though, and I don't think I'd want to do it differently. I got to know myself quite well.

Complicated personalities take a bit longer--there's more to sort out. That doesn't mean I'm any better than other people, but at least I have a very good idea of who I am. I think this might start to get repetitive soon. I just thought you might like to know, being family and all. I'm here. ALL OF ME. Thank God for Bacon (Sir Francis, that is, not the kind we eat at breakfast)!

Well, the sun has gone down and I think its time for dinner. Not much more to say for the moment. The job is going well and I'm thoroughly content. I hope you are.

LOVE, MICHAEL.

P.S. This turned into quite a little letter, didn't it?

NOT A TOTAL WASTE

I often visualize Michael upon his return from Japan, eager to commence his educational research. One of my ultimate goals since his death has been to remember such precious moments, without debilitating emotional pain. Bereavement is expressed in unconscious mechanisms, which cannot always be controlled. Those waves of grief have sometimes seemed completely insurmountable.

Outsiders had surmised that my smiling face and response of, "I'm just fine, thanks," indicated that I had picked up the pieces of my life and returned to "normal". However, Michael's death has changed me forever. I will never return to feeling as I did before Michael's illness and his subsequent death. In the best way that I can, the ongoing experience of grief must be accepted and handled each day. Michael's friends and mine have permitted me to express my grief and alleviated some of my sorrow.

In November, 1992 during a routine business trip to Toronto, a portion of the past became strangely entwined with present events. On the Sunday morning following the conference, Ted and Corey shared brunch with me. We chatted merrily during the meal and then affectionately hugged farewell. Since Bruce was visiting his mother, Corey offered to drive me to the airport.

"Isn't there somewhere you would like to go, before I drop you off at the airport, Maria? We have two extra hours," asked Corey.

I regarded him cautiously and avoided meeting his eyes. I responded, "Yes, Corey. In fact, I'd like to go to the Beaches. I've wanted to visit there ever since...to see where Michael had tried to drown himself..and you pulled him out of the water. Would it upset you, if we went there now?"

Corey contemplated my idea seriously, until a smile slowly transformed his features. He answered, "Yes, Maria. No problem. I love the Beaches. Actually, I go there frequently by myself. The sun seems to have melted this morning's snow and warmed up things. It could be very pleasant to have a walk along the boardwalk. A bit brisk, but enjoyable. Let's go!"

We chatted amiably about many things during the drive and once the car was parked, Corey offered me his arm in a gallant, protective gesture. We walked past the many interesting boutiques and restaurants that had turned the area into a profitable tourist Mecca.

"Now, my car was parked in exactly this same spot on that afternoon. We'll retrace the steps which Mike and I took towards the park area."
"I'm amazed at the number of shops and people, Corey. When I was here as a child these stores did not exist. It has changed drastically, over the years."
"I was unaware that you had lived in Toronto as a youngster. Did you come to the Beaches often?"
"No, Corey. It was reserved as a special family treat. We'd splash in the water, dig in the sand and picnic under the trees."

We straggled through the park's wet, mushy autumn leaves. The Lake Ontario breeze was invigorating and the sun warmed our faces and painted sparkling diamonds on each wavelet that nudged the shoreline. Everywhere we looked, pets and their owners shared a day's hiking. Corey counted fifteen dogs, of various and unknown pedigrees, within an area approximately the size of one city block. On that crisp Sunday afternoon, fresh-air fans of every age and description abounded. As we neared the western edge of the boardwalk, Corey explained,

"This is the exact spot. I hope that it won't upset you, Maria. Mike went into the water there and afterwards, we sat under that large tree and talked for about an hour."
"Here? Right here? How odd," I mused.
"Why? Have you been here before?" Corey put his head to one side and evaluated my reaction.
"As a child, I built castles where the water laps gently against the sand. I have photographs of picnic lunches shared under that very tree. That is the same large smoke stack...and...still, everything is very different."
"Are you upset that Mike would have selected this particular spot?"
"No, Corey, instead it comforts me in some manner just to be here. It's hard to explain, but I have yearned to come here since Mike's death."
"On the anniversary of his death, I walked here alone, Maria. The peacefulness and beauty provided me with some solace on that day, too. So many memories returned."

"I thought about you on that day, Corey. I recalled the assistance you had offered throughout that long, difficult evening, after Michael's death. You're kindness and companionship meant so much to me."

We relaxed and chatted on a bench adjacent to the water and then started towards Corey's parked car. The exertion of the walk and the warmth of the sun had been delightful. As we casually strolled along the boardwalk, we observed a young man shuffling towards us. Unconsciously, we both slowed our steps until we remained transfixed. Alone, he moved steadily, but cautiously, with a slight lurching step. He resolutely pushed his right leg forward with a familiar, swinging gait which was indicative of a partial paralysis on one side. He wore a rust-coloured windbreaker, similar to the one which Michael had brought back from Paris. His spikey, brownish hair was cropped short and he wore round-lensed glasses.

Both Corey and I remained silently stationary, scarcely breathing, as the young man approached us. When he came within an arm's reach, he looked directly into our eyes, smiled gently and nodded as he moved past us. Corey and I turned to each other in helpless amazement. Immediately, Corey put his arm around my shoulder, and hugged me close to his side. My heart beat so fast that I felt its' pounding in my throat. We both blinked away tears and turned to watch the young man's sojourn. As he receded from us, Corey and I searched for an explanation in each others' eyes.

"It was not Mike, Maria. It was NOT Mike. It was just someone who bears a remarkable similarity. You do realize that it was not Mike, don't you?"

"But Corey, he looked and moved so much like him. His gait indicated the same strange, shunting struggle and his clothing was nearly identical. His hair...his glasses...that was a powerful image."

"It was a coincidence. Nothing more. Such things do happen. Maria, Mike is dead. That was definitely not him."

"I realize that. My mind knows that as a truth. And yet..."

"Maria, he will always be with us. It's not abnormal to see someone who reminds us so much of Mike. Many times I have run up the subway steps, chasing after the stranger in a crowd that I would swear is Mike. Once I stand face-to- face with the person,

I am forced to rationalize that Mike is truly dead. Emotions rush over me until I feel almost ill with remorse. It's never easy. You're trembling. Will you be all right?"

"I'm a bit shaken, Corey, but I'm fine. I'm sure glad that you were here with me, when he came along. You've reassured me that my imagination wasn't just in overdrive."

"Other people have had this mystic experience, too, Maria. Identical copies of our loved ones seem to surface from time to time. But we'll have Mike in our thoughts and hearts forever, Maria. We'll always carry a special part of him with us."

Arm in arm, we walked slowly back towards the car. Corey and I were both lost in our own recollections and mindful of one another's emotional upheaval. That "refreshing walk along the boardwalk" had affirmed our own introspective thoughts about Michael. Neither of us felt any need to discuss the experience further. We were comfortable that we had shared those few hours of companionship together, and realized that we could experience another 'deja vu' at some future time. The young man had been so much like Michael, in many respects, that we had been forced to confront his death once again. I was thankful that Corey had been with me during that dramatic encounter. It would have been too petrifying for me, alone. Our trip to the airport was neither sad nor subdued on that sunny, late autumn day. We chatted happily, and waved one another a contented farewell. We still write letters to keep in touch and meet for coffee when I am in the city.

Meanwhile, I continue to deal with grief in stages. Any frustrations which I feel over Mike's death is never consciously allowed to fester, nor used as a negative force to hurt anyone. In particular, I have finally been able to relinquish the futile rage which I felt over Bruce's inability to communicate with Michael during the last two years of his life. I had to let that burden go, and chose not to let those hurts develop into a debilitating bitterness. Michael expected me to use my unconscious energy for positive creative things, instead. He thought that life should be purposeful, and possess meaning. That would have been impossible, if I harbored hurt and anger. I've expressed to Bruce, that while I don't condone his actions at the time that Michael died, I have forgiven him.

In addition, I've discovered how essential it is to forgive myself, and anyone else that may have inadvertently slighted me throughout this traumatic time. Destructive episodes have been set aside, so that hopefully, we can get on with our lives.

The sorrow which Bruce and I experience has become an integral part of our life empiricisms--as much as our marriage, the births of our children and grandchildren, our planned retirements, and our own eventual death. We have been forced to redefine the kind of individuals we intrinsically are, and how we are linked together. Our grief has not followed in subsequent steps, like some agenda, timetable or predictable pattern. We have tasted the shock, anger, depression and isolation that death brings. The nonjudgmental respect and caring provided by friends and loved ones have been treasured gifts. We have fought chronic sleep problems, lack of appetite, thoughts of suicide, inability to function normally, and deep sadness.

When the emotions tend to overtake me, I quietly steal away to my room, light a votive candle and pray for direction and support. The most helpful prayer for me has been the following one, written by Max Ehrmann:

"Let me do my work each day; and if the darkened hours of despair overcome me, may I not forget the strength that comforted me in the desolation of other times.

May I still remember the bright hours that found me walking over the silent hills of my childhood, or dreaming on the margin of the quiet river, when a light glowed within me, and I promised my early God to have courage amid the tempests of the changing years. Spare me from bitterness and from the sharp passions of the unguarded moments. May I not forget that poverty and riches are of the spirit. Though the world know me not, may my thoughts and actions be such as shall keep me friendly with myself.

Lift my eyes from the earth and let me not forget the uses of the stars. Forbid that I should judge others lest I condemn myself. Let me not follow the clamour of the world, but walk calmly in my path.

Give me a few friends who will love me for what I am; and keep ever burning before my vagrant steps the kindly light of hope. And though age and infirmity overtake me, and I come not within sight of the castle of my dreams, teach me still to be thankful for life, and for time's golden memories that are good and sweet; and may the evening's twilight find me gentle still."

There have been continual alterations in our emotions, from one day to the next. We have seen how powerfully the communication of our feelings, without criticism, impacts upon our loved ones. Priorities have continued to evolve and change. Our loss of Michael was more than just a passing depression. Obvious changes within our lives have indicated definite healing. Each day has become more valued, we have accepted more responsibility for the structuring of our future and we have offered more shared affection, while we still live. Michael's demonstrated strength and courage have permitted us to search for meaning and purpose within our own lives.

AFTERTHOUGHTS

(A) Here at last, is a book written to help terminally ill patients and their families face the pain and anguish of impending death.

NOT A TOTAL WASTE is a warm and heartfelt story of a Mother's struggle to assist her son in a fight for life. In her book, Maria Lloyd reveals the very depth of her soul, and lets you feel the pain of her Mother's heart. With daring, she allows you to see the stress that occurs in family relationships when the stark realism of AIDS invades the truth of her son's life. She demonstrates the need for love, compassion, laughter and tears when confronted with death and discrimination. She portrays the importance of respecting the dignity of one's life: by being present to the dying through listening and communicating; by affirming her son's life; by providing a loving presence, so that his aloneness is decreased, on the path to the inevitable.

Maria's actions exemplify the ultimate in Palliative Care. At the same time, she opens a window to the reader, showing a picture of an extremely talented and sensitive young man. NOT A TOTAL WASTE is a stimulating and moving testament of dedication. It is a must for all to read and especially for Health Care Professionals whose privilege it is to care for the dying.

--Janet Fabbro R.N., Director
 Palliative Care Unit

(B) "Do not go gently into that good night,
Rage, rage against the passing of the light."
Dylan Thomas

The AIDS epidemic has taken a devastating toll in Canada and globally from its onset in 1982. Death, suffering and terrible pain have too often been compounded by isolation, loneliness, fear and homophobia. Maria Lloyd's story is a beautiful example of how the love of a mother, as well as the care and compassion of friends and other family members, can so powerfully help to ease the pain and alienation of AIDS. But too many people face this terrible ordeal alone--afraid to tell their families, not that they have AIDS but that they are gay. The lesbian and gay community has demonstrated a tremendous sense of love, community and "traditional family values" in responding to this disease.

Governments have too often been criminally negligent in their response, whether in education, prevention, support, research, or assistance to community based groups on the front lines. As long as governments continue to allow discrimination against lesbians, gay men and bisexuals, people with HIV and AIDS will face not only the pain of the virus but the institutional virus of homophobia, of hatred, of violence. Let us hope that Maria's eloquent story of her son's magnificent life and tragic death will help to prod, if not shame, government leaders to action to effectively fight this epidemic both in Canada and globally.

Michael's friend David said to Maria shortly after Michael's death:

"You owe it to Michael's memory to find new hope, new meaning and purpose in his death. He would want you to harness this experience, value it and put it to some good use."

Michael would, I believe, be very proud to see that his mother has done just what he would have wanted. While Michael did indeed go quietly into that good night, Maria courageously joins her voice in raging, raging against the passing of the light, against this epidemic whose human cost has been incalculable.

--Svend Robinson, MP
House of Commons
Ottawa, ON

ANTI-LESBIAN AND GAY ASSAULTS
A STATISTICAL UPDATE
JUNE 1990 - MAY 1992

253 Reports have been received: 90% from gay men
10% from lesbians

Types of Lesbian and Gay Bashing

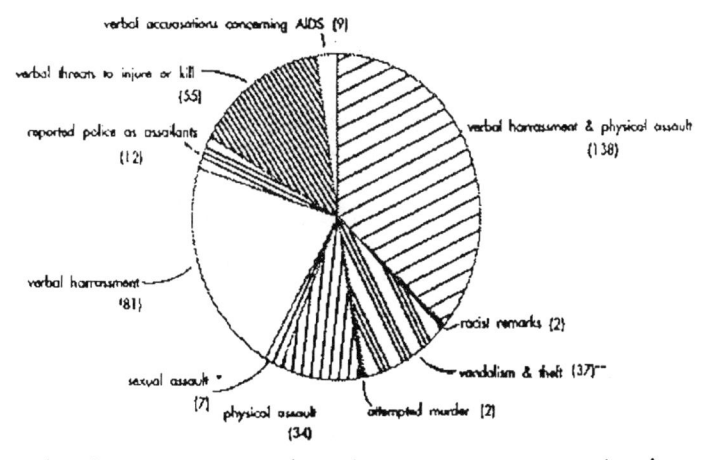

verbal accusations concerning AIDS (9)
verbal threats to injure or kill (55)
reported police as assailants (12)
verbal harrassment & physical assault (138)
verbal harrassment (81)
sexual assault * (7)
physical assault (34)
attempted murder (2)
vandalism & theft (37)**
racist remarks (2)

Data is based on 239 reports to the Hotline. Some items may overlap, for instance, "verbal threats to injure or kill" are also part of "verbal harrassment".

This chart therefore shows the number of occurences of the types of bashing in relation to each other.

* 2 rape, 2 attempted rape, 3 assaults to groin area
** 36 of 37 definitely associated with gay bashing

Weapons

In 68 incidents assailants carried weapons. In some cases more than one weapon was cited. Fists and feet were the most frequent means of causing injury.

AIDS in Ontario

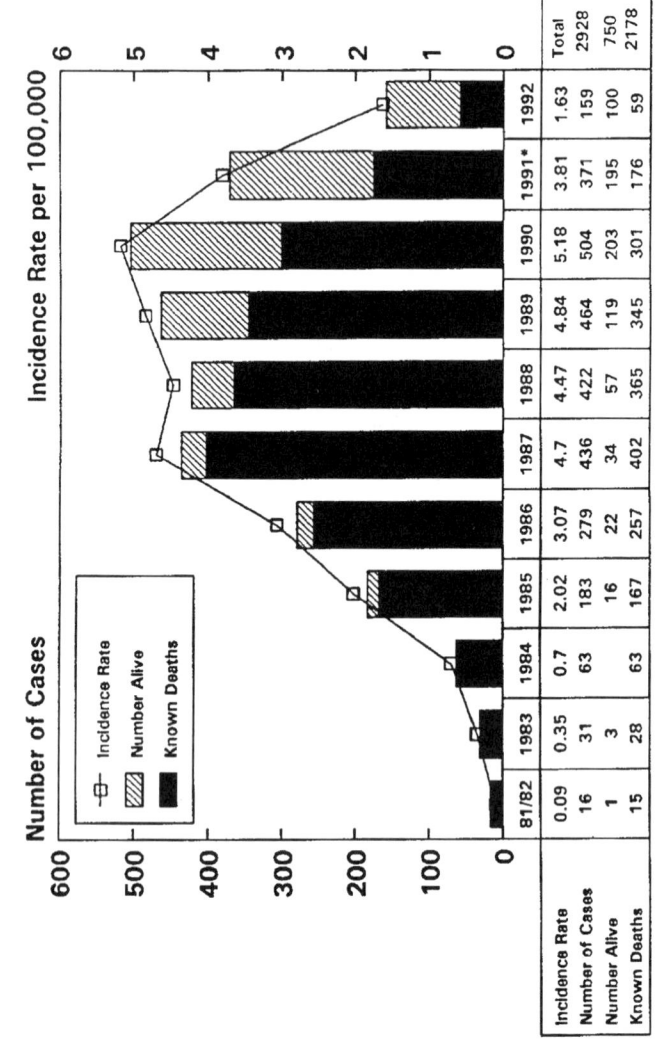

	81/82	1983	1984	1985	1986	1987	1988	1989	1990	1991*	1992	Total
Incidence Rate	0.09	0.35	0.7	2.02	3.07	4.7	4.47	4.84	5.18	3.81	1.63	
Number of Cases	16	31	63	183	279	436	422	464	504	371	159	2928
Number Alive	1	3		16	22	34	57	119	203	195	100	750
Known Deaths	15	28	63	167	257	402	365	345	301	176	59	2178

RUBBERS AND ROMANCE

(From the Brochure "How to Use a Condom" printed in HEALTH Volume 36, Number 7, November/December 1992, pp 100-101. The guide originally appeared in Medical Aspects of Human Sexuality. Every excuse for not using a condom is countered by a logical response.)

I'M ON THE PILL; you don't need a condom.
I'd like to use it anyway. It protects us both from infections we may not realize we have.

I KNOW I'M CLEAN (DISEASE-FREE); I haven't had sex with anyone in X months.
Thanks for telling me. As far as I know, I'm disease-free too. But I'd still like to use a condom since either of us could have an infection and not know it.

I CAN'T FEEL A THING WHEN I WEAR A CONDOM; It's like wearing a raincoat in the shower.
I know there is some loss of sensation and I'm sorry about it. But there are still plenty of sensations left.

I'LL LOSE MY ERECTION by the time I stop and put it on.
Maybe I can help you put it on; that might give you extra sensations, too.

IT'S SO MESSY and smells funny.
Well, sex is that way. But this way we'll be safe.

CONDOMS ARE UNNATURAL, fake, a turn-off.
There's nothing great about genital infections, either. Please let's try to work this out--either give the condom a try or let's look for alternatives.

WHAT ALTERNATIVES did you have in mind?
Just petting and maybe manual stimulation, or we could postpone orgasm, even though I know we both want it.

THIS IS AN INSULT! You seem to think I'm some sort of disease-ridden slut (or giggolo).
I didn't say or imply that. I care about us both and the relationship. In my opinion it's best to use a condom.

NONE OF MY OTHER BOYFRIENDS use a condom. A real man is not afraid.
Please don't compare me to them. A real man cares about the woman he dates, himself, and their relationship.

YOU DIDN'T MAKE JERRY USE A CONDOM when you went out with him.
It disturbs me that you and Jerry talk about me that way. If you believe everything Jerry says, I won't argue with you.

I LOVE YOU! Would I cause infection?
Not intentionally, of course not. But many people don't know they're infected. I feel this is best for both of us at this time.

YOU CARRY A CONDOM AROUND WITH YOU? You were planning to seduce me!
I carry one with me because I care about myself. I made sure I had one with me tonight because I care about us both.

JUST THIS ONCE.
    Once is all it takes.

TASKS TO BE COMPLETED AFTER THE DEATH

Many duties which must be undertaken after the death of a loved one, can make the mourning period even MORE arduous. If an accountant, attorney or close friend could accept some of the following responsibilities, it could assist the bereaved individual.

1. Telephone the doctor, sign the death certificate and establish cremation, funeral or burial arrangements.
2. Make certain that the original will, along with any codicil or separately written notes are provided to the lawyer, and copies are given to all beneficiaries.
3. List any assets or liabilities and determine an inventory of bank accounts and safety deposit boxes.
4. Documents such as wills, power of attorney, living will, death certificate, obituary notice, social insurance number, dates of military service and discharge certification should be located. Sort income tax returns for the last three years. Medical, education and rental expense receipts along with verification of insurance, disability or government payments are needed.
5. Itemize ownership titles to any registered vehicles or loans, with amounts and addresses of the lien holders.
6. List household goods or personal effects valued at more than $1,000.
7. Locate stocks, bonds, mutual fund statements and any broker's statements for the past three years.

8. Bank passbooks, financial statements and cancelled checks for the past three years should be obtained.
9. Life, disability or property insurance policies must be verified, and any needed insurance costs should be paid immediately to protect properties.
10. Pay any debts owed, including medical, hospital or funeral bills.
11. Find all birth, death, marriage, divorce, property settlement and social security certificates.
12. Write confirmation letters immediately to collect death benefits, social securities, injury or accident claims.
13. Services and maintenance contracts such as telephone, rent or utilities must be cancelled or continued.
14. Advise post office of the mail forwarding address.
15. Transfer any household or personal goods and titles for vehicles, to those persons entitled to them.
16. Provide letters or appreciation for any help provided.
17. Contact absent relatives or friends of the deceased by telephone or written letters of notification, regarding the death.

NOT A TOTAL WASTE

MUSIC SOURCES

Borodin, Alexander. Symphony No. 1 in E-Flat Major and Symphony No. 3 in A. Minor. Andrew Davis, Director, Toronto Symphony Orchestra. CBS Inc., YT 42347, 1977.

Lang, K.D. and The Reclines. "Big Big Love", from Absolute Torch and Twang. WEA Music of Canada Ltd., A Warner Communications Company. 92 58774, 1989.

Lee, Peggy. "Hallelujah, I Love Him So" and "Is This All There Is?" from Fever and Other Hits. Capital Records EMI of Canada Limited, 4XL 9095, 1984.

Lennon, John and Paul McCartney. "Strawberry Fields Forever", in The Magical Mystery Tour, Capital Records C248062, 1967.

Lennon, John and Paul McCartney. "I Get By With A Little Help From My Friends", in Serjeant Pepper's Lonely Heart's Club Band. Capital Records, C246442, 1967.

Gould, Glenn. Bach, The Goldberg Variations, BMV988 (Aria and 30 Variations) CBS Inc. Masterworks 40-377779, 1982.

Mitchell, Joni. Both Sides Now (Clouds). Copyright MCMLXVll67, Sequomb Publishing Corporation, Shawnee Press Inc., Delaware, Water Gap, Penn. U.S.A. 18237.

Mozart, Wolfgang Amadeus. No. 1 in D, K. 575, No. 2 in B B Flat, K. 589 and No. 3 in F.K. 590. The String Quartets. Quartetto Italiano. Paolo Borciani & Elisa Pegreffi, violins, Piero Farulli, Viola, Franco Rossi, Violoncello. Philips Classics, 416 419-2, 1971.

Piaf, Edith. "Non, Je Ne Regret Rien" (No Regrets). La Vie En Rose & Other Favorites. Capital Records EMI of Canada Limited, 4XL 57007, 1988.

Pogorelich, Ivo. Ludwig Van Beethoven: Piano Sonata No. 32 in C minor, op. 111, Polydor International GmbH, Hamburg, 3301 036, 1982.

Rogers, Richard and Hammerstein, Oscar. "You'll Never Walk Alone." reprise. Chorus, Samuel Ramey and Barbara Cook in Carousel. Royal Philharmonic Orchestra, Paul Gemignani: Conductor. MCA Records, Inc. MCAC-6209, 1987.

Surnivall, Anthony C. (Arranger) "Amazing Grace". Copyright 1978, Hinshaw Music Inc., P.O. Box 470, Chapel Hill, NC 27514.

Uchida, Mitsuko. Wolfgang Amadeus Mozart, The Complete Piano Sonatas in C, K. 279 to Eine Kleine Gigue in G, K. 574. Philips, 1984, Volumes 1 and 2, 422 116-2, 422 117-2.

NON-TRADITIONAL RESOURCE LISTING ORGANIZATIONS AND SUPPORT GROUPS

Addiction Research Foundation
33 Russell Street
Toronto, ON
M5S 2S1
1-800-387-2916
For assistance or information related to alcohol and other drugs, professional crisis intervention and resources available.

AIDS Education and Public Awareness Program
Canadian Public Health Association
400-1565 Carling Avenue
Ottawa, ON
K1Z 8R1
(613) 725-0376
FAX (613) 725-9826
Information available on all aspects of AIDS education.

AIDS PROJECT--LOS ANGELES
5900 Wilshire Blvd.
Beverly Hills, California 90210
(213) 962-1600
Assistance in education and printed materials about AIDS. A community-based service group providing hands-on care to AIDS patients.

AMFAR--American Foundation for AIDS Research
P.O. Box 17160
Los Angeles, California 90017
(818) 504-2437
American AIDS research Foundation, providing educational material and funding for research on AIDS.

American Association of Suicidology
2459 South Ash Street
Denver, Colorado 80222
(303) 692-0985
Resources for survivors of suicide and literature about the impact of suicide upon the remaining loved ones.

American Civil Liberties Union (ACLU)
132 W. 43rdSt.
New York, NY 10036
(212) 944-9800
Champions the rights of individuals in right-to-die and euthanasia cases. Pamphlets and books available.

American Medical Association (AMA)
535 N. Dearborn St.
Chicago, IL 60610
(312) 645-5000
The AMA is a national professional organization for physicians, with suggested guidelines for euthanasia and hospital policy. Weekly periodicals.

Americans United for Life (AUL)
343 Dearborn St., Suite 1804
Chicago, IL 60604
(312) 789-9494
Public awareness regarding the sacredness of human life.

Bulimia and Anorexia Nervosa Association
3640 Wells Street
Windsor, ON
N9C 1T9
(519) 253-7421
Affiliated with the University of Windsor, some help offered related to diet and AIDS wasting syndrome.

California Medical Association
221 Main St., P.O. Box 7690
San Francisco, CA 94120-7690
(415) 541-0900
Medical ethics, and published paper "Voluntary Active Euthanasia: The Humane and Difnified Death Act."

Center for Death Education and Research
1167 Social Science Building
University of Minnesota
267 19th Avenue S.
Minneapolis, MN 55455
Research into grief and bereavement and responses to death and dying.

Compassionate Friends
P.O. Box 3696
Oak Brook, Illinois 60522-3696
(312) 990-0010
Bereaved parents and professionals are offered education and recent research into the loss of a child.

Compassionate Friends of Canada
685 William Avenue
Winnipeg, Manitoba
R3E 0Z2
(204) 787-2460
Education and research available for bereaved parents.

Concern for Dying
250 West 57th Street
New York, New York 10107
(212) 246-6962
Information on health care and dying, with free Living Will document upon request.

The Elisabeth Kubler-Ross Centre
South Route 616
Head Waters, Virginia 24442
(703) 396-3441
A retreat established by an expert on death and dying, with available educational materials.

Federal Centre for AIDS
301 Elgin Street
Ottaa, ON
KlA 0L3
(613) 957-1772
Information and educational documents related to AIDS.

The Hastings Center
255 Elm Road
Briar Cliff Manor, NY 10510
(914) 762-8500
Support of ethics, public education, treatment of the terminally ill.

Health and Welfare Canada
The National Clearing House on Family Violence
Social Service Programs Branch
Tunney's Pasture
Ottawa, ON
KlA lB5
1-800-267-1291
(613) 957-2936
Educational materials or resource lists related to abuse, family violence, bashing.

Hemlock Society
P.O. Box 11830
Eugene, OR 97440
(503) 342-5748
Membership available, Motto: "Good Life, Good Death". Durable Powr of Attorney for Health Care and Living Will combination provided.

International Anti-Euthanasia Task Force
1205 Pennsylvania Ave.
Golden Valley, MN 55427
(612) 542-3120
An extensive library concerns all aspects of euthanasia. Dedicated to preserving the rights of the terminally ill and to opposing euthanasia.

KIDS HELP Phone Line
1-800-668-6868
A national hotline for children with concerns such as abuse, alcoholism, drug abuse, AIDS.

Make Today Count
P.O. Box 303
Burlington, Iowa 52601
National support group for those experiencing life-threatening disease.

NATIONAL AIDS HOTLINE - USA - 1-800-342-2437
NATIONAL AIDS HOTLINE - CANADA - 1-800-668-2437

National Eating Disorder Information Centre
200 Elizabeth Street, CW1-328
Toronto, ON
M5G 2C4
(416) 340-4156
Telephone, or written information, referral or preventive tools and a newsletter available.

National Funeral Directors Association
11121 West Oklahoma Avenue
Milwaukee, Wisconsin 53227
(414) 541-2500
All funeral resources explained.

National Hospice Organization
Suite 307
1901 North Fort Myer Drive
Arlington, Virginia 22209
(703) 243-5900
Hospice addresses and service organizations offered.

National Organization for Victim Assistance
717 D Street, NW
Washington, D.C. 20004
(202) 393-6682
An advocate group for victims' rights, assistance resources and counselling.

National Self-Help Clearinghouse
Room 620 N
Graduate School and University Center
City Univesity of New York
33 West 42nd Street
New York, New York 10036
(212) 840-1259
Data available on peer support groups of all kinds.

National Right to Life Committee
419 Seventh St. NW, Suite 500
Washington, DC 20004-2293
(202) 626-8800
Ongoing public education programs to oppose euthanasia.
Diane Kent, President

North American Chronic Pain Association
Toronto, Ontario
(416) 793-5230
A support system for persons experiencing any type of pain which has persisted for longer than six months, but that is not associated with on-going tissue destruction.

Parents Without Partners, Inc.
8807 Colesville Road
Silver Spring, Maryland 20910
(301) 588-9354
Crisis intervention, education, social programs for single parents and their children.

Sisters of the Precious Blood
P.O. Box 834
North Bay, ON
PlB 8K1
Prayers offered twenty-four hours a day by religous order for the terminally ill.

Society for the Right to Die
250 West 57th Street
New York, NY 10019
(212) 246-6973

ALSO - 633 Northcliffe Street
Toronto, Ontario
(416) 784-9112
Legislative activity and information on "right to die" legislation. Annual Death with Dignity Legislative Manual and newsletter.

Source of Help in Airing and Resolving Experiences
St. John's Hospital
800 East Carpenter
Springfield, Illinois 62769
(217) 544-6464 (ext. 5275)
A national mutual-help group with publications available pertinent to bereaved parents.

Suicide Information and Education Centre
#201, 1615-10th Ave. S.W.
Calgary, Alberta
T3C-0J7
(403) 245-3900
Materials available for those who have survived suicide, or bereaved families.

The Association for Persons with Severe Handicaps
7010 Roosevelt Way NE
Seattle, WA 98115
(206) 523-8446
Dedicated to providing appropriate services for severely handicapped people, moral considerations for the practice of witholding medical treatment.

The Names Project - The Canadian Memorial Quilt
5224 Blowers Street #206
Halifax, NS
B3J 1J7
(902) 423 9102
The quilt pieces must be six feet by three feet in size, and will be quilted by volunteers before being added to the previous pieces.

The Simple Alternative
197 Sheppart Avenue West
North York, ON
M2N 1M9
(416) 512-1580
The inexpensive procedure for burial, eliminating many cost factors and offering cremation.

They Help Each Other Spiritually
1301 Clark Boulevard
717 Liberty Avenue
Pittsburgh, Pennsylvania 15222
(412) 471-7779
A national group devoted to assisting the widowed person.

The 519 Church Street Community Centre
519 Church Street
Toronto, ON
M4Y 2C9
(416) 392-6874
Newsletter printed providing recent statistics, outlooks related to the Gay and Lesbian community and AIDS. A memorial wall is planned, with names of those who have died from AIDS-related illnesses at Cawthra Park located near the community centre.

Value of Life Committee
637 Cambridge Street
Brighton, MA 02135
(617) 787-4400
Respect for life fostered by educational information. Speakers bureau, library regarding euthanasia, ethics.

GLOSSARY

AIDS
Acquired Immune Deficiency Syndrome
A disease which reduces an affected person's resistance to various types of infections and cancers. A person with AIDS is susceptible to many opportunistic infections and diseases.
AMOEBIASIS
An infection caused by single-celled ameobis microoganisms, often Entamoeba Histolytica, which usually causes severe diarrhea and/or cramping.
ANEMIA
When the blood is deficient in red blood cells, haemoglobin, or in total volume, the anemic condition results.
ASYMPTOMATIC
Infectious organism are present within the body, but no outward symptoms are obvious.
ATYPICAL MYCOBACERTIA
Mycobacterium tubercolosis is the most common mycobacterium which causes human disease (tuberculosis). There are other species which may cause infection in various tissues of immunosuppressed individuals.
BOTULISM
Food poisoning which is life threatening, caused by the botulinus toxin. Human cases are ordinarily found with bacteria found in raw, improperly canned/preserved foods, such as meats and non-acid vegetables. Immediate medical treatment is essential.

CAMPYLOBACTER JEJUNI
The bacterium campylobacter fetus can cause acute illness in the small intestine, resulting in diarrhea, abdominal pain, malaise, fever, nausea and vomiting.
Poultry, raw or unpasteurized milk and milk products can harbour the bacteria.

CANDIDIASIS
Candida albicans causes a yeast-like infection which affects mucus membranes such as skin, nails, and internal organs. This infection may spread throughout the body, and may involve the heart and the central nervous system. Thrush, an oral infection which causes creamy white patches of exudate on inflamed and painful gums is a type of candidiasis. It is also found on the nail beds, axilla, umbilicus, anus, and esophagas. This infection may also be found in the heart, brain lining and spinal cord. It is not uncommon in immune depressed people.

CARCINOGENIC
Inducing the cancerous transformation of cells.

CHEMOTHERAPY
Chemicals or methods that have a toxic effect upon a disease-causing problem.

COLITIS
Inflammation of the large intestine or colon, which is the large intestine terminating at the rectum.

CRYPTOCOCCUS
An infectious disease acquired via the respiratory tract in AIDS patients, primarily in the lungs, and spreading to the meninges (lining of the brain and spinal cord). It can also spread to the kidneys and skin, and is due to the fungus Cryptococcus neoformans. The most common form is meningitis, headache, blurred vision, confusion, depression and agitation.

CRYPTOSPORIDIOSIS
A protozoan parasite located in the intestines of animals can cause this infection. It may be transmitted from person to person, or through direct contact with an infected animal. It lodges in the intestines and causes severe diarrhea. It can lead to prolonged symptoms in AIDS related illnesses, and does not respond to most medications.

CYTOMEGALOVIRUS (CMV)
CMV, related to the herpes family, may occur without symptoms or result in mild flu-like symptoms of aching, fever, mild sore throat, weakness and/or enlarged lymph nodes. Severe CMV

infections can cause hepatitis, mononucleosis, or pneumonia. CMV may cause infections of the eye (retinitis) gastrointestinal tract (colitis) and lungs (pneumonia). CMV is found in body fluids, such as urine, semen, saliva, feces, and perspiration. It includes such infections as CMV Retinities, CMV Gastrointestinal, CMV Colitis, and CMV Pneumonia.
DYSENTERY
Inflammation of the intestines, particularly the colon, causing pain in the abdomen and bloody diarrhea.
EPSTEIN-BARR VIRUS (EBV)
A herpes-like virus causing mononucleosis. It is found in the nose and throat and transferred by kissing. EBV lies dormant in lymph glands and has been associated with cancer of the lymph glands. It is transferred by direct contact, often by kissing.
ENTERIC INFECTIONS
Intestinal infections.
ENCEPHALOPATHY
A disease, previously referred to as dementia, which affects the functions and structures of the brain and central nervous system.
FANSIDAR
Combined pyrimethamine and sulfadoxine, two anti-malarial drugs, used to treat toxoplasmosis and PCP. It may cause a severe, even fatal, skin rash.
GIADIASIS
Intestinal tract infection with a protozoan causing intermittent diarrhea.
GINGIVITIS
Oral gum disease.
GRANULOMATOUS LESION
Lesions which are firm and granular.
HELPER CELLS
Known as T4 cells, these type of T-lymphocyte cells help the B-lymphocytes to produce antibodies.
HEPATITIS
Liver inflammation caused by one of several agents. Jaundice, enlarged liver, fever, fatigue and nausea are common.
HERPES SIMPLEX VIRUS I
A virus which causes cold sores or fever blisters usually around mouth or eyes. It may lie dormant for months or years in nerve tissues and flare up under stress, trauma, infection, or immunosuppression. There are no cures for any herpes viruses.

HERPES SIMPLEX VIRUS II
A virus which causes painful sores on the anus, genitals; can be transmitted to the face or mouth.
HERPES VARICELLA (Zoster Virus)
Chicken pox in children and adult Shingles, consists of very painful blisters on the skin and following nerve pathways.
IMMUNOMODULATING
Therapy which attempts to reconstruct a damaged immune system.
IMMUNOSUPPRESSED
When the body's immune system defenses do not functionproperly as a result of illness or often cancer-fighting drugs.
INTERFERON
An antiviral chemical secreted by an infected cell which serves to strengthen nearby cells.
KAPOSI'S SARCOMA (KS)
A tumour of the walls of blood vessels. This usually appears as pink to purple spots on the skin, but is also found internally or as skin lesions. When major organs are involved, it is rapid and frequently fatal.
LEUKOPENIA
A decrease in the white blood cell count.
MYCOBACTERIUM AVIUM INTERCELLULARE (MAI)
In patients with AIDS, this bacterium caused disease can spread through the blood stream to infect lymph nodes, bone marrow, liver, spleen, spinal fluid, lungs, and intestinal tract. It causes prolonged wasting, fever, fatigue, and enlarged spleen.
NEOPLASTIC DISEASE
Disease caused by uncontrolled, abnormal growth of body tissue.
NODULAR LESION
Raised, hard, mass.
NUCLEOSIDE ANALOG
Synthetic compounds, such as AZT, ddC, and ddI, which suppress replication of HIV.
ONCOGENIC
Creates tumours, especially malignant ones.
OPPORTUNISTIC INFECTIONS
Disease-causing agents normally present within our bodies or the environment which can create diseases when the immune system becomes depressed.

PANCREATITIS
The pancreas gland assists in food digestion, and pancreatitisis is inflammation of the pancreas and can be life-threatening.
PAPILLOMAVIRUS (HPV)
A viral disorder causing warts or nipplelike protrusions.
PNEUMOCYSTIS CARINII PNEUMONIA (PCP)
An airborne lung infection caused by the protozoa Pneumocystis carinii. Once a person develops PCP reoccurrences are common, and the outcome is often fatal when the individual has a weakened immune system.
REMISSION
The abatement of severity or symptoms of a disease.
RETROVIRUS
A group of RNA viruses which cause a variety of diseases in animals.
SALMONELLA
A micro-organism causing fever, diarrhea and/or cramps.
SEROPOSITIVE
The presence of HIV or other bacterial antibodies have been located in a blood sample.
SERONEGATIVE
No HIV or bacterial antibodies found in blood.
SHINGLES
Painful blisters on the skin follow nerve pathways, caused by Herpes Varicella virus.
SHIGELLA
Dysentery can be caused by the micro-organism.
SPUTUM
Mucus ejected from lungs, bronchi, trachea from the mouth.
TOXOPLASMOSIS
The protozoan Toxoplasma Gondii can cause a systemic infection with fever, lymphadenopthy, and lymphocytosis.
VIRUS
Microbes which cause infectious disease within living cells.

(Based upon the HIV/AIDS GLOSSARY from the Aids Committee of Ottawa, 08/01/1991).

REFERENCE SOURCES

Abrahms, J., "Depression versus normal grief following the death of a significant other". In G. Emery, S. Hollon, & R. Bedrosian (Eds.), *New Directions in Cognitive Therapy* (pp. 255-270). New York: Guilford, (1981).

Abramson, L., Seligman, M., & Teasdale, J.,"Learned helplessness in humans: Critique and reformulation". *Journal of Abnormal Psychology*, (1978). 87, 102-109.

Aggleton, P. "HIV/AIDS education in schools: Constraints and possibilities. *Health Education*, (1989). 48 (4), 167-171.

Alvarez, A., *The Savage God: A Study of Suicide*. New York: Penguin Books Ltd., (1971).

Anthony, S., *The Child's Discovery of Death*. New York: Harcourt, (1940).

Aries, P., *Western Attitudes Toward Death: From the Middle Ages to the Present*. Baltimore: John Hopkins University Press, (1974).

Arthur, B., & Kemme, M. L., "Bereavement in Childhood," *Journal of Child Psychology and Psychiatry*, (1964), 37-49.

Averill, J., "Grief: Its Nature and Significance". *Psychological Bulletin*. (1968), 70, 721-748.

Barnard, C., *Good Life/Good Death*. Englewood Cliffs, NJ: Prentice-Hall, (1980).

Barrows, Marjorie, Editor. *Treasures of Love and Inspiration.* (New York, NY: Galahad Books, Inc., 1986).

Bascue, L.O., "Counselor experiences with client death concerns". *Rehabilitation Counselling Bulletin.* (1977), 21:37
Batchelor, Walter F.,"AIDS: A Public Health and Psychological Emergency". *American Psychologist.* (1984).
Battigan, M. G., "Giving Death a Helping Hand". *The Journal of the Canadian Medical Association.* (1991), Vol. 144, No.3, 358-359.
Beck, A., Ward, C., Mendelson, M., Mock, J., & Erbaugh, J., "An inventory for measuring depression". *Archives of General Psychiatry.* (1961), 4, 561-571.
Becker, E., *The Denial of Death.* New York: The Free Press, (1973).
Behnke, M., Reiss, J., Neimeyer, G., "Grief responses of pediatric house officers to a patient's death". *Death Studies.* 1987), LL, 169-176.
Bowlby, J., *Attachment and Loss.* (Vol.3), New York: Basic Books, (1980).
Bridges, W., *A Year in the Life.* New York: Bantam Books Inc., (1982).
Brooks-Gunn, J., Boyer, C.B., and Hein, K. "Preventing HIV infection and AIDS in children and adolescents: Behavioral research and intervention strategies. (1988). *American Psychologist* (1988), 43, 958-963.
Brown, L.K., Fritz, G.K. and Barone, V.J. "Impact of AIDS education on junior and senior high school students". *Journal of Adolescent Health Care* (1989), 10, 386-392.
Bugental, J., & Bugental, E., "A fate worse than death: The fear of changing". *Psychotherapy.* (1984), 21, 543-549.
Burda, D. & Powills, S. "AIDS: A time Bomb at Hospitals' Door". *Hospitals.* (January, 1986).
Capron, A.M., "Ironies and tensions in feeding the dying". *Hastings Center Report.* (1984), 14:5 32-35.
Caputo, L. "Dual Diagnosis: AIDS and Addiction". *Social Work.* (July/August, 1985).
Cates, W. and Rauh, J.L. "Adolescents and sexually transmitted disease: An expanding problem". *Journal of Adolescent Health Care.* (1985),. 6, 257-261.
Celan, Paul. Poems of Paul Celan: Translated, with an Introduction by Michael Hamburger (New York: Persea Books, 1988).
Center for Disease Control. "HIV-related beliefs and behaviors among high school students". *MMRE* (1988), 717-721.

Center for Disease Control. *HIV/AIDS Survaillance Report.* (1991).
Childers, P., & Wimmer, M., "The Concept of Death in Early Childhood," *Child Development.* (1971), 42, 705-712.
Christ, G.H., & Weiner, L.S. "Psychosocial Issues in AIDS". In Devita, V.T. Jr., Hellman S., & Rosenberg, S.A. *AIDS - Etiology, Diagnosis, Treatment, & Prevention.* New York: J.B. Lippencott Co. (1985).
Choron, J., *Death and Western Thought.* New York: Collier, (1976).
Cimbolic, P., & Jobes, D.A. (Eds.), *Youth Suicide: Issues, Assessment, and Intervention.* Springfield, Ill.: C.C. Thomas. (1990).
Clark, E.J., Fritz, J.M., Rieker, P.P., Kutscher, A.H., and Bendiksen, R.A., (Editors): *Clinical Sociological Perspectives and Illness and Loss.* Philidelphia, PA: The Charles Press, Publishers, (1990).
Clarke, D. "AIDS education: A community approach". *Health Education.* (1988), 47 (4), 85-89.
Coates, T.J. "Strategies for modifying sexual behavior for primary and secondary prevention of HIV disease". *Journal of Consulting and Clinical Psychology,* (1990), 58, 57-59.
Coates, T.J., Temoshok, L., & Mandel, J. "Psychosocial Research is Essential to Understanding & Treating AIDS". *American Psychologist.* Vol. 39, No. 11, (November, 1984), pp 1309-14.
Conroy, R. J., "Critical incident stress debriefing". *F.B.I. Law Enforcement Bulletin.* (1990). 59:2, 67-69.
Corr, C.A., & Corr, D. (Eds.), *Hospice Approaches to Pediatric Care.* New York: Springer, (1985).
Corr, C.A., & and McNeil, J. (Eds.), *Adolescence and Death.* New York: Springer, (1986).
Cullinan, A.C., "Trauma: Causes, effects, and interventions. *Illness, Crises and Loss* (1991), 1:2, 41-48.
Curran, W.J., "Defining appropriate medical care: providing nutrients and hydration for the dying". *New England Journal of Medicine.* (1985), 313, 940-942.
Curtis, H., Lawrence, C., and Tripp, J. "Teenage sexuality: implications for controlling AIDS. *Archives of Disease in Childhood.* (1989), 64, 1240-1245.
Crase, D., and Hamrick, M., "Death Education Within Health Education". *Health Education,* (1990) Vol. 21, No.3, May/June, 44-48.
Cronella, A.C. "The Person Behind the Disease". *Nursing '85.* Vol. 15, No. 9, (September 1985).

Danto, B.L., and Kutscher, M.L., (Editors): *Suicide and Bereavement.* New York: Arno Press/A New York Times Company, (1978), pp. 269.
DeBellis, R., Goldberg, I.K., Kutscher, A.H., Blitzer, A., Gerber, I., and Tretter, P., (Editors): *Medical Care of the Dying Patient.* New York: Arno Press/A New York Times Company, (1982).
DeBellis, R., Kutscher, A.H., Goldberg, M.R., Cherico, D.J., Klagsbrun, S.C., and Prichard, E.R., (Editors): *Women and Loss.* New York: Praeger Publishers, (1985), pp. 222.
DeBellis, R., Marcus, E.R., Kutscher, A.H., Smith-Torres, C., and Barrett, V.W., and Siegel, M.E., (Editors): *Suffering: Psychological and Social Aspects in Loss, Grief and Care.* New York, NY: Haworth Press, (1986).
Dempsey, D., "Learning how to die", *The New York Times Magazine.* (1971), 11, 60.
Dempsey, D., Carse, J.P., Donovan, C., Kutscher, A.H., Cherico, D.J., and Cohen, M., (Editors): *Death, the Press and the Public: Presentations To, For, and By the Media and Other Professionals.* New York: Arno Press/A New York Times Company, (1981).
DeSpelder, L.A. & Strickland, A.L. *The Last Dance: Encountering Death and Dying.* (1987), Mountainview: Mayfield Publishing.
Deuchar, N. "AIDS in New York City with Particular Reference to the Psycho-Social Aspects". *British Journal of Psychiatry.* Issue 145, (1984), pp 612-619.
Dick, H.M., Roye, D.R. Jr., Buschman, P.R., Kutscher, A.H., Rubenstein, B., and Forstenzer, F.K., (Editors): *Dying and Disabled Children: Dealing with Loss and Grief.* New York, NY: The Haworth Press, Inc., (1989).
DiClemente, F.J. Zorn, J., and Temoshok, L. "Adolescents and AIDS: A survey of knowledge,attitudes and beliefs about AIDS in San Francisco. *American Journal of Public Health.* (1986), 76, 1443-1445.
DiClemente, F.J. "Prevention of human immunodeficiency virus infection among adolescents: The interplay of health education and public polilcy in the development of school based AIDS education programs". *AIDS Education and Prevention* (1989), 1 (1), 70-78.
Dilley, J.W. "Treatment Interventions & Approaches to Care of Patients with Acquired Immune Deficiency Syndrome". In Nichols, S.E., & Ostrow, D.G., editors.

Dilley, J.W., Ochitill, H.N., Perl, M., & Volberding, P.A. "Findings in Psychiatric Consultations with Patients with Acquired Immune Deficiency Syndrome". *American Journal of Psychiatry.* Vol. 142, No. 1, (January 1985).
Donlow, J., Walcott, D.L., Gottlieb, M.S., Landsverk, J. "Psychosocial Aspects of AIDS and AIDS-Related Complex: A Pilot Study". *Journal of Psychosocial Oncology.* Vol. 3, No. 2, (Summer 1985).
Downey, J.A., Reidel, G., and Kutscher, A.H., (Editors): *Bereavement of Physical Disability, Commitment to Life, Health and Function.* New York: Arno Press/A New York Times Company, (1982).
Dresser, R.S., Boisaubin, E.V.,"Ethics, law and nutritional support", *Archives on Internal Medicine.* (1985), 145, 122-124.
Durkheim, E., *Suicide.* New York: MacMillan Publishing Co., (1951).
Earle, A.M., Argondizzo, N.T., and Kutscher, A.H., (Editors): *The Nurse as Caregiver for the Terminal Patient and His Family.* New York: Columbia University Press, (1976), pp. 243.
Eliot, T., "Bereavement as a problem for family research and technique", *The Family.* (1930), 11, 114-115.
Ellis, A., "The rational-emotive approach to thanatology". In H. Sobel (Ed.), *Behavior and therapy in terminal care: A humanistic approach.* (1981). (pp. 151-176). Cambridge, MA: Ballinger.
Feifel, G., *Something After Death.* Leeds: John Blackburn Limited, (1974).
Feifel, H., *The Meaning of Death.* Toronto: McGraw-Hill Book Company, Inc., (1959).
Feifel, H., "Death and dying in modern America", *Death Education.* (1977), 1, 5-9.
Ferrara, A.J. "My Personal Experience with AIDS". *American Psychologist.* (November, 1984).
Firestone, R.W., and Seidan, R.H., "Suicide and the Continuum of Self-Destructive Behaviour". *Journal of American College Health.* (1990), Vol. 238, No.5, March, 207-213.
Fleming J., & Altschul, S., "Activation of Mourning and Growth by Psychoanalysis," *International Journal of Psychoanalysis.* (1963), 44, 419-432.
Fleming, S. J., "Parental Social Adjustment After the Death a Child." In preparation, (1984).

Fleming, S. J., & Robinson, P., "The application of cognitive therapy to the bereaved". In M. Vallis & J. Howes (Eds.), *The challenge of cognitive therapy: Applications to non-traditional populations*. New York: Plenum, (1991).
Forstein, M. "AIDS Anxiety in the 'Worried Well'". In Nichols, S., & Ostrow, D. *Psychiatric Implications of Acquired Immune Deficiency Syndrome*. Washington, D.C.: American Psychiatric Press, Inc., (1984).
Frank, Arthur. At the Will of the Body (New York: Houghton Mifflin, 1987).
Freud, S., "Inhibitions, Symptoms and Anxiety." (1926), in *The Standard Edition of Complete Psychological Works of Sigmund Freud*, translated by J. Strachey, 24 vols. London: Hogarth Press, (1959), Vol. 20, pp. 87-172.
Fulton, R., *Death and Identity*. New York: Wiley, (1965).
Fulton, R., *Death, Grief and Bereavement*. New York: Arno Press, (1977).
Fulton, R., *Death and Dying: Challenge and Change*. Massachusetts: Addison-Wesley Publishing, (1987).
Gibran, K., On death, In *The Prophet*. New York: Alfred A. Knopf, (1923).
Gallagher, E., (Editor): *Will I Live Another Day Before I Die?* New York, NY: Foundation of Thanatology, (1989).
Galt, M., Gillies, P., and Wilson, K. "Surveying knowledge and attitudes towards AIDS in young adults; Just 19". *Health Education*, (1989), 48 (4), 162-166.
Gibran, Kahil. *The Prophet*. (New York, NY: Alfred A. Knops, 1923).
Gillies, P. "Educating teenagers about AIDS: Recent developments in the USA. *Health Education*, (1988), 47(4), 162-166.
Glaser, B. G., & Strauss, A. L., *Time for Dying*. Chicago: Aldine, (1968).
Glaser, B. G., & Strauss, A. L., *Awareness of Dying*. Chicago: Aldine, (1965).
Goldberg, I.K., Kutscher, A.H., and Malitz, S., (Editors): *Pain, Anxiety and Grief: pharmacotherapeutic care of the dying patient and the bereaved*. New York: Columbia University Press, (1986), pp. 228.
Gonsiorek, J.C. *A Guide to Psychotherapy with Gay & Lesbian Clients*. New York: Harrington Park Press, (1985).
Gorer, G., *Death, Grief and Mourning*. Garden City, New York: Doubleday, (1965).

Gorer, G., "The pornography of death", *Modern Writing*. New York: Berkely, (1956).
Gottlieb, M.S., Schoroff, S.O. and Schanker, H.M. "Pnuemocytis carinii pneumonia and mucosal candidiasis in previously healthy homosexual men: evidence of a new acquired cellular immunodeficiency". *New England Journal of Medicine*. (1981), 305, 1425-1431.
Goulden, T., Todd, P., Hay, R., & Dykes, J. "AIDS and Community Support Services. Understanding and Management of Psychological Needs". *The Medical Journal of Australia*. Vol. 141, No. 9, (October 27, 1984).
Grof, S., and Halifax, J., *The Human Encounter with Death*. New York: E.P. Dutton, (1978).
Grollman, A., *Concerning Death: A Practical Guide for the Living*. Boston: Beacon, (1974).
Grollman, A., *Explaining Death to Children*. Boston: Beacon Press, (1967).
Gullo, S.V., Patterson, P.R., Schowalter, J.E., Tallmer, M., Kutscher, A.H., and Buschman, P., (Editors): *Death and Children: A Guide for Educators, Parents, and Caregivers*. New York: Tappan Press, (1985), pp. 208.
Gunther, J., *Death Be Not Proud*. New York: Harper & Row, (1949).
Hamilton, M., and Reid, H., *A Hospice Handbook: A New Way to Care for the Dying*. Grand Rapids, Michigan: W.B. Erdmans Publishing Company, (1980).
Hardt, D.V., *Death the Final Fronteir*. New Jersey: Prentice-Hall, Inc., (1979).
Hausman, K. "Treating Victims of AIDS Poses Challenge to Psychiatrists". *Psychiatric News*. Vol. XVIII, No. 15, August 5, 1983.
Hendin, D., *Death As A Fact Of Life*. New York: W.W. Norton Publishers, (1973).
Hetrick, E.S., Stein, T.S., editors. "Innovations in Psychotherapy with Homosexuals". *American Psychiatric Press, Inc.* Washington, D.C., (1984).
Hidalgo, H., Paterson, T.L., Woodman, N.J., editors. "Lesbian & Gay Issues: A Resource Manual for Social Workers". *National Association of Social Workers*. Silver Spring, Maryland, (1985).
Hinton, J., *Dying*. Baltimore, Md.: Penguin, (1972).

Hingson, R., Strunin, L., Berlin, B.M., and Heerson, T. "Beliefs and AIDS, use of alcohol and drugs, and unprotected sex among Massachusetts adolescents". *American Journal of Public Health* (1990), 80, 295-299.

Hodgkinson, P. "Abnormal grief: The problem of therapy", *Journal of Child Psychology and Psychiatry*. (1964), 37-49.

Jackson, E., *Telling a Child about Death*. New York: Hawthorn Books Inc., (1965).

Jackson, E., *Understanding Grief*. Nashville: Abingdon, (1957).

Janke, J. "Dealing with AIDS and the adolescent population". *Nurse Practitioner*, (1989), 14 (11), 35-41.

Joseph, J.G., Emmons, C., Kessler, R.C., Worman, C.B., O'Brian, K., Hocker, W.T., Schaefer, C. "Coping With the Threat of AIDS: An Approach to Psychosocial Assessment". *American Psychologist*. Vol. 39, No. 11, (November 1984).

Kalish, R., *Death, Grief and Caring Relationships*. Monterey, California: Brooks/Cole Publishers, (1985).

Kane, A.C. and Hogan, J.D. "Death anxiety in physicians: defensive style, medical specialty, and exposure to death. (1985), Omega, 16, 11-21.

Kaplan, H. and Sadock, B. eds. *Comprehensive Textbook of Psychiatry*. (1991), Baltimore: Williams and Wilkens.

Kastenbaum, R., "We covered death today." *Death Education*. (1977), 1, 85-90.

Kastenbaum, R., *Death, Society and Human Experience*. St. Louis: Mosby, (1977).

Kastenbaum, R., "Childhood: the kingdom where creatures die". *Journal of Clinical Psychology*. (1974), 13, 85-97.

Kastenbaum, R., "The realm of death: an emerging area in psychological research". *Journal of Human Relations*. (1977), 3, 11-17.

Kavanaugh, R., *Facing Death*. Baltimore, Md.: Penguin, (1972).

Kay, W.J., Nieburg, H., Kutscher, A.H., Grey, R.E., and Fundin. C., (Editors): *Pet Loss and Human Bereavement*. Ames, Iowa: Iowa State University Press, (1984), pp. 198.

Keller, S.E., Barlett, J.A., Schleifer, S.J., Johnson, R.L., Pinner, E. and Delaney, B. "HIV-relevant sexual behavior among a healthy inner-city heterosexual population in an endemic area of HIV". *Journal of Adolescent Health Care*. (1991), 12, 44-48.

Kirby, D., Harvey, P.D., Claussenius, D., and Novar, M. "A direct mailing to teenage males about conom use: Its impact on knowledge, attitudes and sexual behavior". *Family Planning Perspectives*, (1989), 21 (1), 12-18.

Klagsburn, F., *Youth and Suicide: Too Young To Die.* Boston: Houghton Mifflin Company, (1976).

Klass, C., *Parental Grief: Solace and Resolution.* New York: Springer, (1988).

Kluge, Eike-Henner Ph.D., "Euthanasia and related taboos". *The Journal of the Canadian Medical Association.* (1991), Vol. 144, No.3, 359-360.

Knapp, R. J., *Beyond Endurance: When a Child Dies.* New York: Schocken, (1986).

Knott, J.E., "Death education for all". *Dying: Facing the Facts.* Washington, DC: Hemisphere Publishing, (1979).

Koop, C.E. *Surgeon General's Report on Acquired Immunodeficiency Syndrome.* (1986), Washington, D.C.: US Public Health Service.

Kooperman, C., Rotherman-Borus, M.J., Henderson, R., Bradley, J.S. and Hunter, J. "Assessment of knowledge of AIDS and beliefs about AIDS prevention among adolescents. *AIDS Education and Prevention*, (1990), 2(1), 58-69.

Krasnik, A., and Wangel, M. "AIDS and Danish adolescents: Knowledge, attitudes and behavior relevant to the prevention of HIV infection". *Danish Medical Bulletin* (1990), 37(3), 275-279.

Krell, R., & Rabkin, L., "The Effects of Sibling Death on the Surviving Child: A Family Perspective". *Family Process.* (1979), 471-477.

Kubler-Ross, E., *Death: The Final Stage of Growth.* New York: Prentice-Hall, (1975).

Kubler-Ross, E., *Questions and Answers on Death and Dying.* New York: The MacMillan Company, (1974).

Kubler-Ross, E., *On Death and Dying.* New York: MacMillan Publishing Co., Inc., (1969).

Kubler-Ross, E., and Warshaw, M., *To Live Until We Say Goodbye.* Englewood Cliffs, N.J.: Prentice-Hall, (1978).

Kushner, H. S., *When Bad Things Happen to Good People.* New York: Schochen, (1981).

Kutscher, A.H., Bess, S., Klagsburn, S.C., Siegel, M.E., Cherico, D.J., Kutscher, L.G., Peretz, D., and Selder, F.E., (Editors): *For the Bereaved: The Road to Recovery.* Philadelphia, PA: The Charles Press, Publishers, (1990).

Kutscher, A.H., and Goldberg, M.R., (Editors): *Caring for the Dying Patient and His Family.* New York: Health Sciences Publishing Corporation, (1973).

Kutscher, A.H., and Kutscher, L.G., (Editors): *For the Bereaved.* 125 essays. New York: Fredrick Fell, Inc., (1971).

Kutscher, A.H., Kutscher, L.G., and Jaffe, L., (Editors): *Dialogues: the Dying and the Living.* New York: Arno Press/A New York Times Company, (1978), pp. 275.

Kutscher A.H., Peretz, D., Klagsbrun, S., Cherico, D.J., and Kutscher, L.G., (Editors): *For the Bereaved--But Not to Lose: A Book of Comfort.* (revised edition). New York: Arno Press/ A New York Times Company, (1980).

LaGrand, L. *Coping With Separation and Loss As A Young Adult.* (1986), Springfield, Illinois: Charles C. Thomas.

Lamerton, R., *Care of the Dying.* Middlesex, England: Penguin Books, Ltd., (1980).

Lampl-de-Groot, J., "Mourning in a Six-Year-Old Girl," *Psychoanalytic Study of the Child.* (1976), 31, 273-281.

Lampke, R.S., Fishman, M., Kutscher, A.H., Grossi, C.E., Halporn, R., Liegner, L.M., and Chachkes, E., (Editors): *Prespectives on the AIDS Crisis: Thanatological Aspects.* New York, NY: Foundation of Thanatology, (1989).

Latimer, Elizabeth M.D., "Caring for Seriously Ill and Dying Patient: The Philosophy and Ethics". *The Journal of the Canadian Medical Association.* (1991), Vol. 144, No. 7, 859-863.

Laughlin, L.," Suicide: the ultimate gamble". *Teen Generation.* (1982), 42, 13-15.

Lennon, M. C., & Martin, J. L., "The Influence of Social Support on AIDS - Related Grief Reaction Among Gay Men". *Social Science Medicine.* (1990), Vol. 31, No. 4, 477-484.

Lerner, G., *A Death of One's Own.* New York: Harper Colophon Books, (1987).

Leshan, E., *Learning to Say Good-by.* New York: MacMillan, (1976).

Lewis, C. S., *A Grief Observed.* London: Faber, (1961).

Lief, H., Fisher, W.A., Furstenberg, N. "Human sexuality with respect to AIDS and HIV infection". *Sieccan Newsletter* (1990), 25 (3), 8-25.

Lifton, R., and Olsen, E., *Living and Dying.* New York: Bantam Books, (1975).

Linn, E., *I know how you feel....Avoiding the cliches of grief.* Cary, Ill.: Publisher's Mark, (1986).
Longman, A., Lindstrom, B., and Clark, M., Prelimanary evaluation of bereavement experiences in a hospice program, *The Hospice Journal.* (1989), 5, 34.
Lopez, D.J., & Getzel, G.S. Helping Gay AIDS Patients in Crisis. *Social Casework.* (September, 1984).
Lukas, C., & Seiden, H. M., *Silent Grief: Living in the Wake of Suicide.* New York: Charles Scribner's Sons, (1987).
Margolis, O.S., Kutscher, A.H., Marcus, E.R., Rather, H.C., Pine, V.R., Seeland, I.B., and Cherico, D.J., (Editors): *Grief and the Loss of an Adult Child.* New York: Praeger Publishers, (1988), pp. 193.
Margolis, O.S., Reather, H.C., Kutscher, A.H., Volk, R.J., Goldberg, I.K., and Cherico, D.J., (Editors): *Grief and the Meaning of the Funeral.* New York: Arno Press/A New York Times Company, (1975), pp. 270.
Margolis, O.S., Reather, H.C., Kutscher, A.H., Powers, J.B., Seeland, I.B., DeBellis, R., and Cherico, D.J., (Editors): *Acute Grief--Counselling the Bereaved.* New York: Columbia University Press, (1981), pp. 269.
Martin, J.L., Vance, C.S. "Behavioral and Psychosocial Factors in AIDS". *American Psychologist.* Vol. 39, No. 11, (November, 1984).
Massey, D. "Teaching about AIDS in school". *Health Education.* (1987), 46 (2), 27-36.
McConville, B. J., Boag, L. C., & Purohit, A. P., "Mourning Process in Children of Varying Ages". *Canadian Psychiatric Association Journal.* (1970), 15, 253-255.
Meyer, M.F. "The Gay Patient in Psychological Context: Some Thought". *B.C. Medical Journal.* Vol. 27, No. 6, (June, 1985).
Miller, D. & Gunn, J. "Psychological Support & Counselling for Patients with Acquired Immune Deficiency Syndrome (AIDS)". *Genitourinary Medicine.* Vol. 61, No. 4, (August, 1985).
Miller, T.E., Booraem, C., Flowers, J.V., Iverson, A.E. "Changes in knowledge, attitudes and behavior as a result of a community-based AIDS prevention program". *AIDS Education and Prevention,* (1990), 2 (1), 12-23.
Mitford, J., *The American Way of Death.* New York: Simon and Schuster, (1978).
Moriarity, D. M. (Ed.), *The Loss of Loved Ones.* Springfield, Il: Charles C Thomas, (1967).

Morin, S.F., & Batchelor, W.F. "Responding to the Crisis of Aids." *Public Health Reports.* Vol. 99, (January/Feruary, 1984).

Morin, S.F., & Charles, K.A., Maylon, A.K. "The Psychological Impact of AIDS on Gay Men". *American Psychologist.* Vol. 39, No. 11, (November, 1984).

Moses, A.E. & Hawkins, R.O. *Counselling Lesbian Women and Gay Men: A Life Issues Approach.* St. Louis: The C.V. Mosby Company, (1985).

Mott, F.L., and Haurin, R.J. "Linkages between sexual activity and alcohol and drug use among American adolescents". *Family Planning Perspectives* (1988), 20 (3) 128-136.

Nader, P.R., Wexler, D.B., Patterson, T.L., McKusick, L., and Coates, T. "Comparison of beliefs about AIDS among urban, suburban, incarcerated, and gay adolescents". *Journal of Adolescent Health CareTp.* (1989), 10, 413-418.

Nagy, M., "The Child's Theories Concerning Death". *Journal of Genetic Psychology,* (1948), 73, 3-27.

Navia, B.A., Jordan, B.P., Price, R.W. "The AIDS Dementia Complex; l Clinical Features". *Annals of Neurology.* Vol. 19, (1986), pp 517-24.

Naifeh, S. W., & Smith, G. W., *Why Can't Men Open Up?* New York: C.N. Potter, (1984).

Newell, M.M., Naylor, H.H., Marcus, B., Kutscher, A.H., Cherico, D.J., and Seeland, I.B., (Editors): *The Role of the Volunteer in the Care of the Terminal Patient and the Family.* New York: Arno Press/A New York Times Company, (1981).

Nichols, S.E. "Psychiatric Aspects of AIDS". *Psychosomatics.* Vol. 24, No. 12, (December, 1983).

Nichols, S.E. "Social & Support Groups for Patients with Acquired Immune Deficiency Syndrome". *American Psychiatric Press, Inc.* Washington, D.C.,(1984).

Nichols, S.E. & Ostrow, D.G. "Psychiatric Implications of Acquired Immune Deficiency Syndrome". *American Psychiatric Press, Inc.* Washington, D.C., (1984).

Nouwen, H. J. M., *A Letter of Consolation.* San Francisco: Harper and Row, (1982).

O'Connor, B., Cherico, D.J., and Kutscher, A.H., (Editors): *The Role of the Minister in Caring for the Dying Patient and the Bereaved.* New York: Arno Press/A New York Times Company, (1978).

Osis, K. (Ph.D.), and Erlendur Haraldsson, (Ph.D)., *What They Saw: At the Hour of Death.* New York: Avon Books, (1977).
Overstreet, B., *Understanding Fear in Ourselves and in Others.* New York: The MacMillan Company, (1970).
Papadatos, C., & Papadatou, D. (Eds.), *Children and Death.* New York: Hemisphere, (1989).
Parkes, C. M., *Bereavement.* New York: International Universities Press, (1971).
Parkes, C. M., *Bereavement: Studies of Grief in Adult Life.* (2nd ed.), New York: Penguin Books, (1986).
Parry, J.K. (Ed.), *Social Work Practice with the Terminally Ill.* Springfield, Ill.: C.C. Thomas. (1990).
Peck, S., *The Road Less Travelled.* New York: Simon and Shuster, (1978).
Pine, V.R., Kutscher A.H., Peretz, D., Slater, R.C., DeBellis, R., Volk, R.J., and Cherico, D.J., (Editors): *Acute Grief and the Funeral.* Springfield, IL: Charles C. Thomas, Publisher, (1976), pp. 321.
Pine, V.R., Margolis, O.S., Doka, K., Kutscher, A.H., Scheafer, D.J., Siegel, M.E., and Cherico, D.J., (Editors): *Unrecognized and Unsanctioned Grief: the Nature and Counselling of Unacknowledged Loss.* Chicago, IL: Charles C. Thomas, Publishers, (1990).
Prohaska, T.R., Albrecht, G., Levy, J.A., Surgue, N., and Kim, J.A. "Determinants of self-perceived risk for AIDS". *Journal of Health and Social Behavior,* (1990), 31, 384-394.
Prunkl P., & Berry, R., *Death Week.* New York. Hemisphere Publishing, (1989).
Psychiatric Implications of Acquired Immune Deficiency Syndrome. *American Psychiatric Press,* In. Washington D.C., (1984).
Quint, J.C., *The Nurse and the Dying Patient.* New York: Macmillan Publishing Co., (1967).
Rando, T., *Grief, Dying and Death.* Champaign, Illinois: Research Press, (1984).
Rando, T., *Parental Loss of a Child.* Champaign, Ill.: Research Press, (1986).
Rando, T. A., *Grieving: How to Go On Living When Someone You Love Dies.* Toronto: D.C. Heath and Co., (1988).
Raphael, B. A., *Bereavement Counseling: A Multidisciplinary Handbook.* Westport, Conneticut: Greenwood Press, (1980).

Reeves, R. Jr, Neale R.E., and Kutscher A.H., (Editors): *Pastoral Care of the Dying and Bereaved - Selected Readings.* New York: Health Sciences Publishing Corporation, (1973).
Rickert, V.I., Jay, M.S., and Gottlief, A. "Effects of a peer counselled AIDS education program on knowledge, attitudes, and satisfaction of adolescents". *Journal of Adolescent Health Care,* (1991), 12, 38-43.
Richards, H., *Death and After: What Will Really Happen?* London: Fount Paperbacks, (1980).
Robinson, L. A., "Social skills training program for adult caregivers". *Advances in Nursing Science.* (1988), 10, 159-72.
Royal Bank of Canada. "Facing up to death". *The Royal Bank Letter.* (1982), 63, 3.
Russel, O., *Freedom to Die.* New York: Human Sciences Press, (1975).
Rynearson, E.K. "Psychological effects of unnatural dying on bereavement". *Psychiatric Annals.* (1986), 16, 272-275.
Sanders, C., *Grief: The Mourning After.* New York: Wiley, (1989).
Schiff, H. S., *The Bereaved Parent.* New York: Crown, (1977).
Schneider, J. *Stress, Loss and Grief.* (1984), Baltimore: University Park Press.
Schoenberg, B., Carr, A.C., Peretz, D., Kutscher, A.H., and Goldberg I.K., (Editors): *Anticipatory Grief.* New York: Columbia University Press, (1974), pp. 381.
Schoenberg, B., Gerber, I., Wiener, A., Kutscher, A.H., Peretz, D., and Carr, A.C., (Editors): *Breavement: Its Psychosocial Aspects.* New York: Columbia University Press, (1975), pp. 368.
Schoenberg, R., Goldberg, R.S, editors, with D.A. Shore. *With Compassion Toward Some: Homosexuality & Social Work in America.* New York: Harrington Park Press, (l985).
Schowalter, J.E., Buschman, P., Patterson, P.R., Kutscher, A.H., Tallmer, M., and Stevenson, R.G., (Editors): *Children and Death: Perspectives from Birth through Adolescence.* New York: Praeger Publishers, (1987).
Schowalter, J.E., Patterson, P.R., Tallmer, M., Kutscher, A.H., Gullo, S.V., and Peretz, D., (Editors): *The Child and Death.* New York: Columbia University Press, (1983), pp. 352.
Schultz, R., *The Psychology of Death, Dying and Bereavement.* Reading, Mass.: Addison-Wesley, (1978).
Seeland, I.B., Klagsbrun, S.C., DeBellis, R., Kutscher, A.H., Avellanet, C., and Dennis, J., (Editors): *The Final 48 Hours: Observations on the Last Days of Life.* Philadelphia, PA: The Charles Press Publishers, (1991).

Shneidman, E., *Voices on Death*. New York: Harper and Row, (1980).
Shneidman, E., Death: *Current Perspectives*. California: Mayfield, (1976).
Skinner, B., *Beyond Freedom and Dignity*. New York: Alfred A. Knopf, (1972).
Smith, B., *Dear Gift of Life*. Pennsylvania: Pendle Hill, (1965).
Stanford, G., and Perry, D., *Death Out of the Closet*. New York: Bantam Books, Inc., (1976).
Stein, A.J. "Debriefing: The aftermath of a tragedy". (1991). Paper presented at the 13th Annual Conference of The Association for Death Education and Counseling. Duluth, Minnesota.
Sterobe, W., & Stroebe, M.S., *Bereavement and Health*. Cambridge University Press, (1987).
Sudnow, D., *Passing On: The Social Organization of Death*. Engelwood Cliffs, New Jersey: Prentice Hall, (1967).
Suszycki, L.H., Abramson, M., Kutscher, A.H., Prichard,E . R ., and Fischer, D., (Editors): *Social Work and Terminal Care*. New York: Praeger Publishers, (1984).
Sy, F.S., Richter, A., and Copello, A.G. "Innovative educational strategies and recommendations for AIDS prevention and control". *AIDS Education and Prevention* (1989), 1 (1) 53-56.
Tallmer, M., Clason, C., Lampke, R.F., Kutscher, A.H., Braun, E., and Selder, F.E., (Editors): *HIV Positive: Perspectives on Counselling*. Philadelphia, PA: The Charles Press, Publishers, (1991).
Tallmer, M., DeSanctis, P., Bullard, B.G., Kutscher, A.H., Roberts, M.S., and Patterson, P.R., (Editors): *Sexuality and Life-threatening Illness*. Springfield, Il: Charles C. Thomas Publishers, (1984).
Tagliaferre, Lewis, & Harbaugh, Gary, L., *Recovery From a Loss: A Personalized Guide to the Grieving Process*. Deerfield Beach, Florida: Health Communications, (1990).
Taylor, R., *The Will to Live: Selected Writings of Arthur Schopenhauer*. New York: Fredrick Unger Publishing Co., (1975).
Temes, R., *Living With an Empty Chair*. New York: Irvington Publishers, (1980).
Turnbull, R. (Ed.), *Terminal Care*. New York: Hemisphere Publishing, (1986).
Veninga, R.L., *A Gift of Hope*. New York: Ballantine, (1985).

Walker, G. "Crises-care in critical incident debriefing". *Death Studies.* (1990), 14, 121-133.
Watson, W., and Maxwell,R., *Human Age and Dying.* New York: St. Martin's Press, (1977).
Weininger, O.,"Young Children's Concepts of Dying and Dead". *Psychological Reports.* (1979), 44, 395-407.
Weisman, C.S., Nathanson, C.A., Ensminger, M., Teitelbaum, M.A., Robinson, J.C., and Plichta, A.S. "AIDS knowledge, perceived risk and prevention among adolescent clients of a family planning clinic". *Family Planning Perspectives,* (1989), 21 (5), 213-215.
Wessels, D.T., Kuscher, A.H., Seeland, I.B., Selder, F.E., Cherico, D.J., and Clark, E.J., (Editors): *Professional Burnout in Medicine and the Helping Professions.* New York, NY: The Haworth Press, Inc., (1989).
White, D.G., Phillips, K.C., Pitts, M., Clifford, J.R. and Davies, M.N. "Adolescents' perception of AIDSP. *Health Education,* (1988), 47 (4), 117-119.
Wolf, S.G., Kutscher, A.H., and Clark, E.J., (Editors): *The Role of the Community Hospital in Dealing with Life-Threatening Disease and Bereavement.* New York: Archives of the Foundation of Thanathology, (1980).
Wolf, S.G. Jr., Torpie, R.J., Kutscher, A.H., Sheridan, P., Durie, B., and Peretz, D., (Editors): *Caregiving in the Community Hospital: for the Terminally Ill and the Bereaved.* New York: Arno Press/A New York Times Company, (1982).
Woodman, N.J. & Lenna, H.R. *Counselling with Gay Men and Women.* San Francisco: Jossey-Bass Publishers, (1980).
Worden, J. W., *Grief Counselling and Grief Therapy.* New York: Springer. (1982).
Wortman, C., & Silver, R., "The myths of coping with loss". *Journal of Consulting and Clinical Psychology.* 57, 349-357, (1989).
Wylie, B. J., *Beginnings.* Toronto: McCelland and Stewart, (1977).
Zelnik, M. and Shah, F.K. "First intercourse among young Americans". *Family Planning Perspectives* (1983), 15 (2), 64-70.

How HIV virus spreads

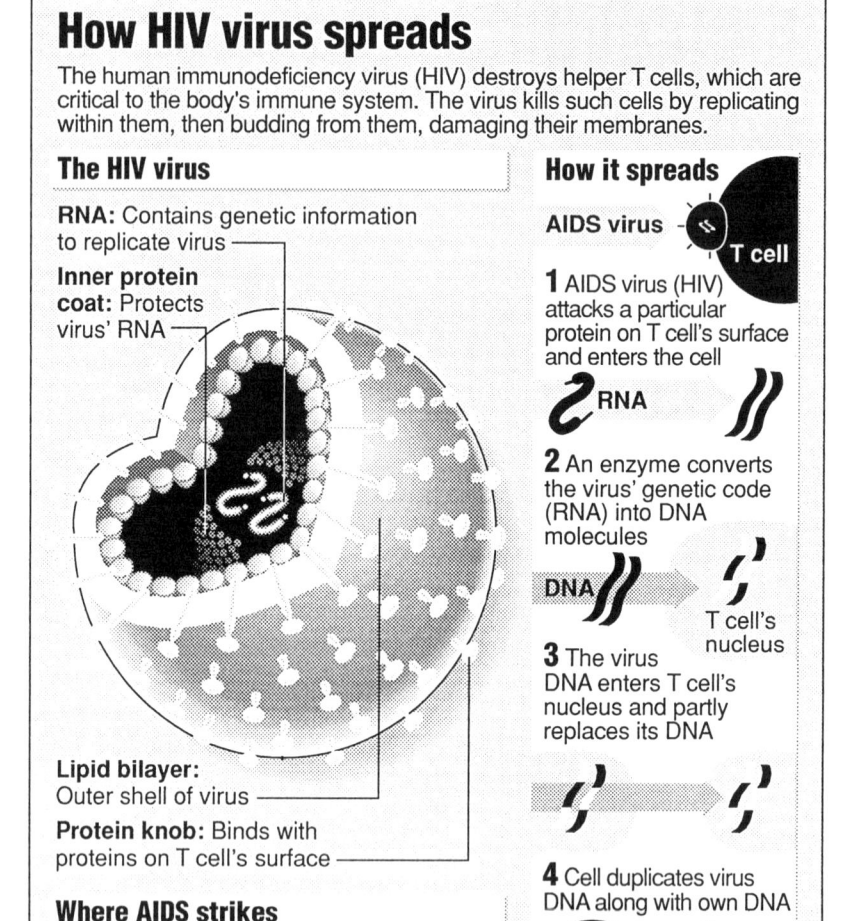

The human immunodeficiency virus (HIV) destroys helper T cells, which are critical to the body's immune system. The virus kills such cells by replicating within them, then budding from them, damaging their membranes.

The HIV virus

RNA: Contains genetic information to replicate virus

Inner protein coat: Protects virus' RNA

Lipid bilayer: Outer shell of virus

Protein knob: Binds with proteins on T cell's surface

Where AIDS strikes

- Brain
- Lymph nodes
- Thymus gland
- Lung
- Lymphocytes in blood, semen, vaginal fluid
- Skin
- Bone marrow
- Colon, duodenum, rectum

SOURCES: Department of Health and Human Services, Public Health Service, Centers for Disease Control, Scientific American, news reports

How it spreads

AIDS virus → T cell

1 AIDS virus (HIV) attacks a particular protein on T cell's surface and enters the cell

2 An enzyme converts the virus' genetic code (RNA) into DNA molecules

3 The virus DNA enters T cell's nucleus and partly replaces its DNA

4 Cell duplicates virus DNA along with own DNA

5 Under guidance of DNA and RNA made from it, cell produces new proteins; some are AIDS proteins

6 Proteins assemble into new AIDS virus, which escapes through cell membrane, out into body

11/30/92   Knight-Ridder Tribune/RON CODDINGTON

NOT A TOTAL WASTE

World AIDS cases

The number of reported AIDS cases is dramatically lower than the estimates because of under reporting, delays in reporting and under diagnosis.

Estimated AIDS and HIV cases

AIDS — 2 million
HIV infections — 9-11 million

Reported AIDS cases

Cumulative number of cases reported to the World Health Organization as of March 1992:
In thousands

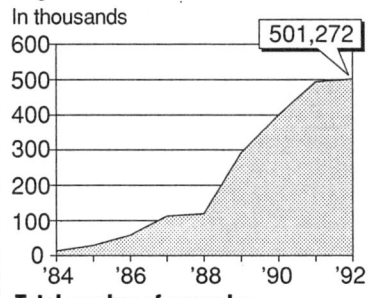

'84	13,135
'85	28,578
'86	57,642
'87	112,806
'88	119,136
'89	291,351
'90	400,223
'91	493,872
'92	501,272

Continent	Cases
Africa	152463
Americas	277042
Asia	1552
Europe	66545
Oceania	3670

Total number of cases by continent, 1992:

Continent	Cases
Americas	277,000
Africa	150,000
Europe	67,000
Oceania	3,700
Asia	1,600

SOURCE: World Health Organization

11/30/92 Knight-Ridder Tribune/C. GAFFNEY

CATEGORY: NATIONAL NEWS
SUBJECT: SUB World AIDS cases
ARTIST: Cordelia Gaffney
ORIGIN: KRT
TYPE: Freehand
SIZE: 1 column
ENTERED: 11/30/92
REVISED:
STORY SLUG:

© Copyright 1992 Knight-Ridder Tribune, Inc.
Reprint with permission only. The credit "Knight-Ridder Tribune" or "KRT" must appear with all uses of this graphic image.

EXCERPTS FROM DAVID'S LETTER, SENT TO MARIA- -SHORTLY AFTER MICHAEL'S DEATH

...In the end, Michael was forced to watch, helpless, as the worst and most malignant of our nightmares waged war on his body; and yet he, as with thousands of other brave men before him, faced that nightmare with a courage, dignity and personal freedom that was, in the true sense of the word, awesome...

...Yet he was not seeking comfort. He was seeking understanding...Michael was fascinated by three things: puppets, architecture and the way children learn. He wanted to understand the structures of power and how they could be used, both for good and evil. For a child, a puppet can be a great source of comfort, solace and learning. For an adult, it can describe the techniques by which we seek to destroy others. A building can be either a home or a prison; it all depends on who holds the key...

...The road that Michael took was not an easy one...He did manage to develop an enormous strength that came from knowing that he never flinched from life...Michael did not succumb to trivial comforts at the expense of his own integrity. He would not deny who he was and what was happening to him. If he must die of a hideous plague, then he would do it on his own terms--and he did...His acute rationalism and his analytical tools allowed him to maintain his dignity in the face of an almost unbelievable assault. What was the source of that courage, that human wisdom?

...Shortly before he died, Michael bought that wonderful silk shirt. It was a funny, vibrant pastiche of colour. I think it summarized much of what he had lived for and something of what he had come to know. It was a celebration of spirit--an exaltation of larks--a joyful recognition that he was the master of his own spirit...Death may be merely an absence of constraints, a great gaping nothingness. But like Michael's shirt--what a bright, glorious, shimmering, nothingness!

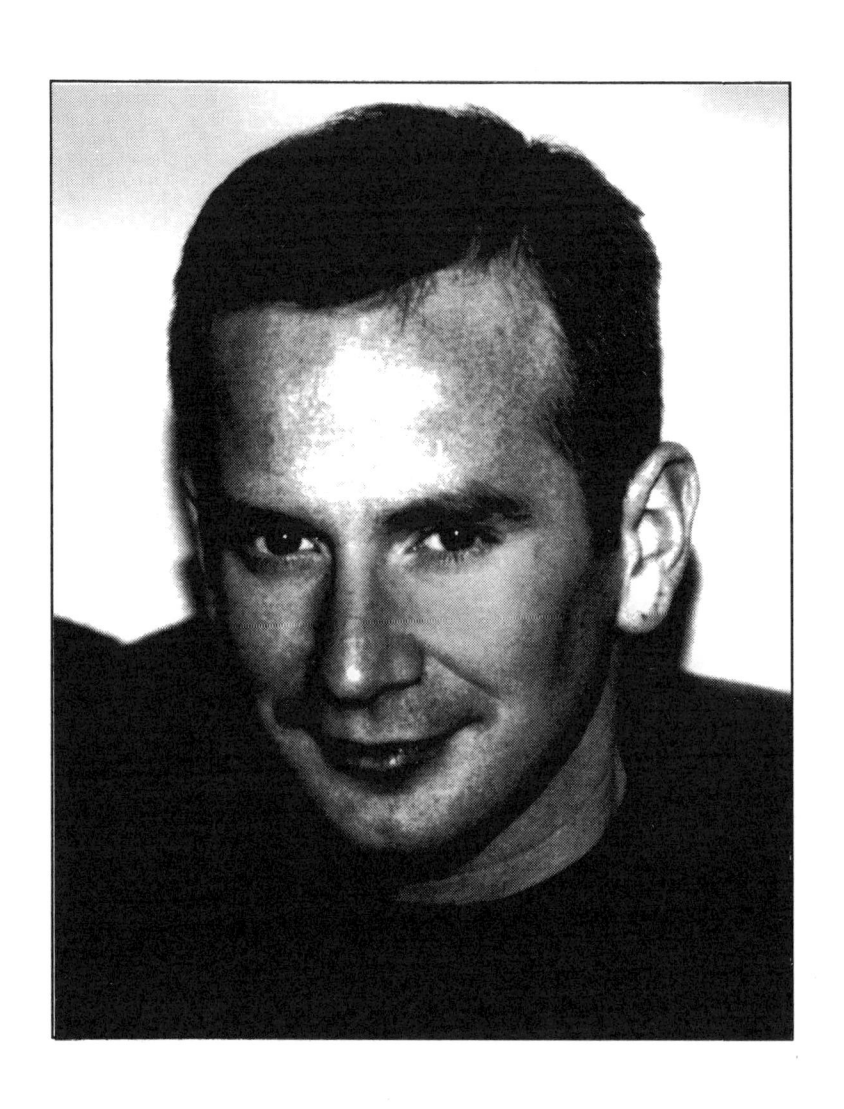

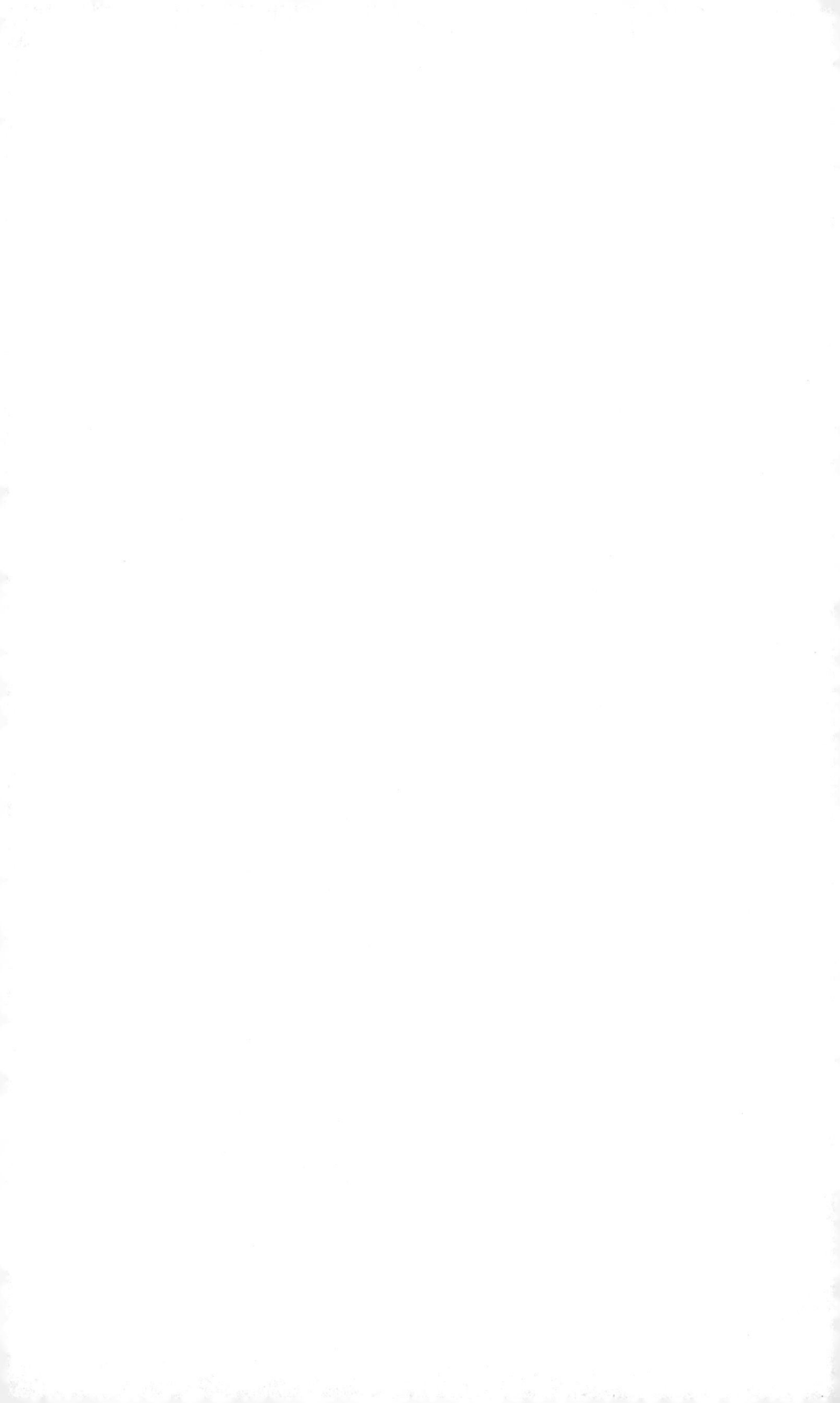